THE ONLY
DIET EXERCISE & WEIGHT-LOSS
BOOK
YOU WILL EVER NEED TO READ

Dedication:

To my clients, family and friends, and to all, the people that I have had the privilege to meet within this wonderful industry. Being able to assist people in changing their lives is a rewarding feeling that words can hardly describe! Thank you everybody, for being a part of my journey. Always remember: Celebrate your Mind, Body, and Life.

I hope you enjoy this incredible book.

Steve Gallagher

Start Here X

Based solely on evidence-based weight-loss and exercise science, my book continues to receive accolades from Primary Care Physicians, Registered Dietitians, and Informed Health Professionals. The Fitness & Weight-loss Industry earns billions annually, selling empty promises and false hope to uninformed consumers. Let's face it, the words "Fast", "Easy", and "Effortless" will often make otherwise intelligent people, act stupidly. This book is filled with the easy-to-understand explanations of the topics people ask about most, or get wrong, most often. You can expect to easily trouble-shoot your own exercise-routine or diet, to understand why it is failing to produce the results you are desire. More importantly, you will be able to make "results" suddenly begin to happen.

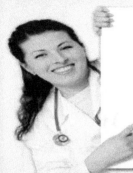

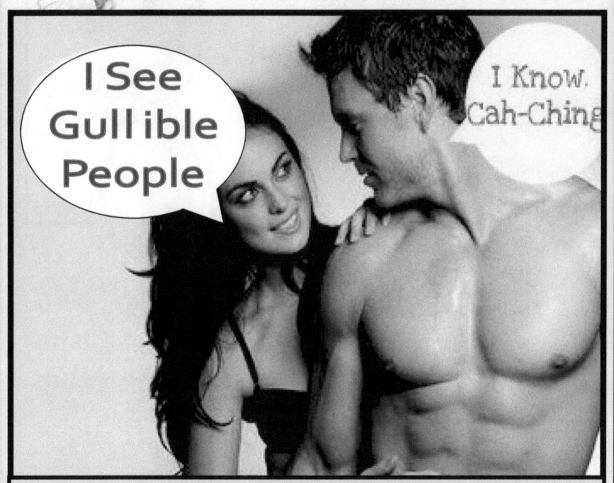

Chapter 1

For Starters...

Learn to Recognize

Lies & "BS"

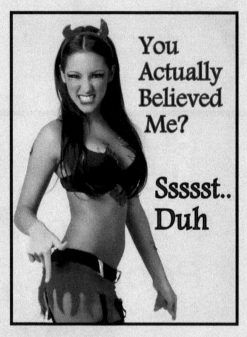

You Actually Believed Me?

Ssssst.. Duh

Chapter 2

Eating & Weight-loss Ahhh.... Now I Get It!

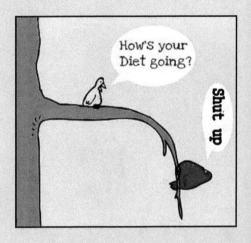

Chapter 3

EXERCISE RESULTS Ahhh... Now I Get It!

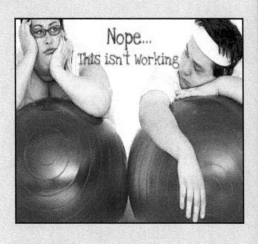

Chapter 4

Things Even "Smart People" STILL Get Wrong

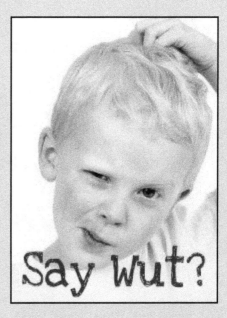

Say wut?

Chapter 5

Q&A, FYI's N' Stuff

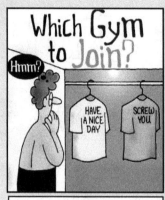

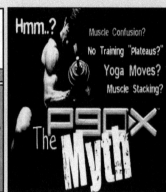

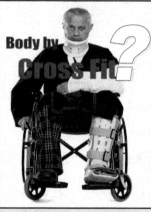

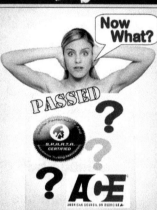

Chapter 1

For Starters...
Learn to Recognize
Lies, Myths,
& "BS"

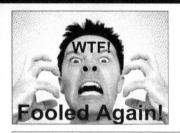

WTF!
Fooled Again!

Why We Fall For Total "BS"

Why do we believe most of the "BS" we are told about dieting, exercise, and weight-loss? It's probably because the magic words, ***"Fast, Easy, and Effortless"***, can often make otherwise intelligent people act totally stupid. Exercise and Weight-loss Marketers are more focused on gimmicks - the things they think you'll buy - than on sound exercise and weight-loss principles. The sources we rely on for credible information are often just BS Artist trying to make a buck off of our ignorance. As you already know, they can make it sound so appealing. It usually goes something like this...

"Amazing Results-Fast!"
"Ripped In 30-Days!"
"It's So Easy!"
"Melt Belly-Fat"
"Limited Time Only"
"Scientifically Proven"
"Before-and-After Photos"
"Testimonials by Celebrities"
"Patented Formula"
"Secret Ingredients"
"Not Sold in Stores"
"FDA Approved"
"Unbelievably Easy"...Etc.

What they're really saying is:
"This Stuff is Bull Crap...
We just hope you're stupid enough to BUY IT"

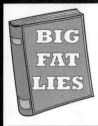 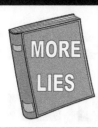

New Diets & Diet Books

There is virtually a type of "Diet" for every letter of the alphabet.
Try to say them all in one breath...

**Alkaline diet - Atkins diet - Best Bet Diet - Beverly Hills diet - Blood Type Diet
Body for Life diet - Breatharian diet - Buddhist diet - Cabbage Soup Diet - Cookie diet
Crash diet - Detox diet - Diabetic diet Dr. Hay diet - Eat Clean Diet - Earth Diet - Endemic diet
Elemental diet - Elimination diet - Fit for Life diet - Flexitarian diet Food combining diet
F-plan diet - Fruitarian diet - Gerson diet - Gluten-free diet - Casein-free diet
Graham diet - Grapefruit diet Hacker's diet - Hay diet - Halal diet - Hallelujah diet
High-protein diet - Healthy Six diet - Inuit diet - Israeli Army diet - Jenny Craig diet
Joel Fuhrman diet - Junk food diet - Juice diet - Kosher diet - Ketogenic diet
Lacto vegetarianism diet - Liquid diet - Low-carbohydrate diet - Low-fat diet
Low glycemic index diet - Low-protein diet - Low sodium diet - Macrobiotic diet - McDougall diet
- Medifast Diet - Mediterranean diet - Montignac diet - Natural Foods diet - Negative calorie diet
Nutrisystems diet - Okinawa diet - Omnivore diet - Organic food diet - Ovo-lacto vegetarian diet
Paleo diet - Perricone diet - Pescetarian diet Plant-based diet Pritikin diet - Rastafarian diet
Raw diet - Scarsdale Medical Diet - Shangri-La Diet - Slimming World diet - Slim Fast diet
Smart For Life Sonoma diet South Beach diet - Spark People diet - Stallman diet
Subway diet - Vegan diet Vegetarian diet - Weight Down diet - Weight Watchers diet
Western pattern diet, and the Zone diet.** ...I think you get the picture!

Although Diet Book Authors try to convince you otherwise, the truth is, Nutritional Science hasn't changed much over the years. For example, Scientists discovered the first vitamin about one-hundred years ago. It took them less-than-a-year to discover the rest. Although nutritional science is complicated on a cellular-level, practically everything you need to know about losing-weight could be learned in one day. Year-after-year, new Diet Book Authors claim that "they" alone have unlocked the secret to fast and easy weight-loss. Of course, they're full of BS. Want proof? Walk into any bookstore and go right to the "Diet Book" Section. Every book you see will soon be replaced by another book making "new" claims for the upcoming year. 6 months from now, chances are you will not see any of today's books on those same book shelves. There will always be new "Diet Books" written by new authors, again hoping to convince you that they possess the secret to weight-loss. **The only "loss" is usually the loss of your money.**

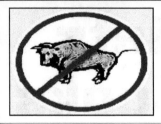 # Not-So-Scientific Research

"Research Proves" "Studies Show"
My Question: What research? What Studies? Don't Be Fooled!

The thing you must always consider regarding "Research" is who's conducting it and do they have a stake in the outcome. For example; Diet and Fitness magazines are filled with "ghost-written" articles. (Meaning, your favorite celebrity didn't write the article even though their name is on it as "written by"). These articles are notorious for naming ambiguous research in an attempt to validate their "pitch". In other words, attempting to get you to buy whatever bogus crap they're selling. It usually sounds something like this:

1 - "Research shows that…"(What research are they talking about?)

2 - "Scientific-Research proves…" ("Everything" is "scientific". I just threw a football and hit my pal Joey in the head - The Law of Physics - Duh!)

3 - "Studies have shown…"(Again, "WHAT" studies are they citing?)

4 - "Research shows Weightlifters who use "Nitro-Creatine" are 75% stronger!" (75% stronger than who, 5th-Graders? Also, who buys "Nitro-Creatine? Weightlifters do! So weightlifters are 75% stronger than non-weightlifters. This makes sense, but has nothing to do with Nitro-Creatine.)

One of my favorites: **"Recent taste-test research revealed 9 out of 10 Cola-drinkers prefer Pepsi over Coke!"** (Do you REALLY think "Coke" sponsored that "taste-test?") Just for fun, the next time you hear a pitch for a product, every time the word "research" or "studies" is used, replace it (in your mind) with the word "bullsh*t". It's funnier than watching a TV Sit-Com.

Bottom Line: Most credible scientific research is conducted by Major Universities, and then, reported on in peer-reviewed science journals. It is written in technical language which is complicated and confusing to a lay-person. Truly "Geek" stuff. When a commercial company (selling a product) conducts it's own research, or sponsors outside research. It's a pretty safe bet that the researcher's findings will shine favorably on that company's product. Wow, what a surprise!

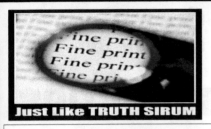
Just Like TRUTH SIRUM

The "Fine-Print" NEVER Lies

The Final Insult to Your Intelligence; The Fine Print

Ever wonder WHY the fine-print at the bottom of TV Ads is so tiny n' small? Answer: It's because it's usually the "only" thing in the entire ad, that is not a lie. The next time you see a TV-ad trying to sell a new idiotic way to lose weight or get fit, instead of listening to the lies they are spewing, look immediately at the "fine print" on the bottom of the screen...Unfortunately, it will probably look like this...Don't even try to read it.

JJFIJFGROJIGJOIP IOOREIJGR OIJIJRO IJOI IKCOIIE TRFCTV POE OIVI OOVV OIIORFJKV UI9HVIJV OIVN OINJVOI OIEFVBIJN OIPFJVJV FDIJVIJ OPFJVKJV FIV FJKVNOI RIVJJIV VOIJ OV

For the most part, advertisers are pretty much able say whatever they want to pitch their products. However, most bogus claims and bullshit lies can only be made if a "disclaimer" or "disclosure" is included in the advertisement.

Here's a few examples: of the "Claim" and then, the "Fine Print"...

"I lost 20 pounds in just 4 weeks using *"Melt-Away Fat Burners"*

These results are not "typical". Reduced calorie eating and regular exercise.

"After watching *Ivan-the-Idiot's Workout Video,* I developed rock-solid Abs just in time to hit the beach this summer. - Thanks Ivan!"

The actors in this advertisement are compensated for their testimonial.

"When I want to pack on extra muscle in the off-season, I reach for a *"Mega-Muscle Protein Drinks"*...what's in your bottle?"

These statements have not been reviewed by the FDA and have not been proven to be accurate or true. This product is a food supplement, and is not intended to replace food in

The "Fine-Print" always tells the truth...
BS Artists just hope you WON'T read it.

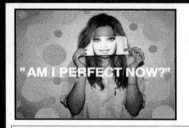
"AM I PERFECT NOW?"

Movie Stars & TV Personalities

We really don't have to spend much time here - it's really simple. TV Fitness Experts are really Salespeople and "paid" Spokespersons. They come into your living room trying to get rich selling you shit you don't need. Who are they? There are 4 basic types:

1) A washed-up TV star trying to cash-in on "face recognition".
2) A famous-person's (Oprah's) Personal Trainer. Instant "credibility".
3) An attractive Fitness Model or Bodybuilder Star, selling "You can look like me!"
4) A person the "Industry" is paying to be a Spokesperson based solely on their "looks", "believability", or "likeability" factor. In other words, they don't have to possess any (real) qualifications - and they usually don't! Here's an off-the-top-of-my-head list of some of the most notable "TV" Fitness Experts. Every one of them fits into one of the before-mentioned categories. Today, many are either gone from the public-eye after making millions, selling their Exercise Tapes, Workout Machines, or Special Weight-loss Programs. ALL of them will soon be replaced by the "next" TV Expert looking to make their big pay-day!

Billy Blanks (Tae Bow Videos)
Jillian Michaels (TV Personal Trainer)
Richard Simmons (Sweatin' to the Oldies)
Body by Jake (TV Personal Trainer)
Tony Little (The "Gazelle Glider" Exercise Machine)
Jennilee Webb (Buns of Steel Videos)
Denise Austin (TV Exercise Guru)
Kathy Smith (Exercise Video Queen)
Susan Powter (Stop the Insanity Program)
Christie Brinkley (The Total Gym Machine)
Susan Somers (The Thigh Master)
Chuck Norris (The Total Gym Machine)
Shawn T ("Insanity" by Beachbody)
...the latest "Expert" - Tony Horton (P90X)

Remember: Scientific breakthroughs are not "For Sale" on TV-Infomercials. No "TV" Expert has EVER changed the laws of Exercise-Science with their "Revolutionary" new product or exercise machine. - none ever will. You are going to encounter many more of these BS artists in your lifetime. Next time, just laugh - and then change the channel.

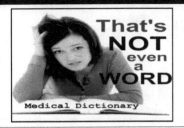

That's NOT even a WORD

Medical Dictionary

"Supplement Ads?" LIES, LIES, LIES...

SUPPLEMENT Companies DON'T Really Care IF Their Products Even WORK! That's NOT Even Their Objective. You MUST understand that Supplement Manufacturers DO NOT try to create products that works. Instead, they try to create products that they think you will buy. Big difference. The Company's decision to introducing a "new" product has nothing to do with a product's effectiveness - It has everything to do with PROFITABILITY! Supplement Companies continue to make billions of dollars selling you products that they know DO NOT produce the results they promise. "Fat-Burners" and "Metabolism-Boosters" - Yeah, RIGHT! So, why do we purchase the bogus-products that promise super-fast weight-loss or incredible muscle-growth? Answer: Because we are desperate and impatient. The good-for-nothing products you need to lookout for are usually easy to spot. Just look for anything that uses these words on their product label:

Mega - Blast - Turbo - Super - Nitro - Ultra - Ripped - Pro - Anabolic Torched Inferno - Furnace - Lean - Extreme - Insanity - Energized Pumped - Juiced X-treme - Super charged - Maxx - Shredded - Etc.

Here's a typical "Metabolism-Boosting" product-claim:
"Rev Your Metabolism and TORCH Calories with Our TURBO Fat-Burning Shake!"
This is a perfect example of a Supplement Ad misleading you by twisting the ACTUAL truth. Whenever we eat food, it goes through a digestive-process. "Digestion" itself is a "Metabolism". The body has many metabolisms. And, like all other metabolic-processes (another word for metabolism) it takes calories to carry-out the task of digesting food. Scientist call this the "Thermic-Effect" of food. In other words, to process calories, your body must use calories to do it. However, the calories needed for digestion will NEVER out-number the calories in the food being digested. For example, when you eat 500-calories of "anything" your body may burn 50-calories to digest it. But, so what. It doesn't negate the other 450-calories. So yes, eating "any" food will increase your body's overall metabolism. But, only because digestion is occurring, which is in itself a metabolism. Supplement Manufacturers trying to sell "Fat-Burners" actually twist this science, and it comes out sounding like this: "Drinking XYZ Fat-Burning Shake causes the body to burn calories!" Well, Duh!

B-E-W-A-R-E of The "Pretty People"

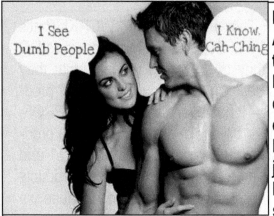

EYE-CANDY and PERSONAL TRAINING Will ALWAYS be a Profitable Marketing Combination. Unfortunately, it can Also Be a Mirage. Personal Trainers - the good ones - are hired to coach their clients through safe, effective, and evidence-based exercise programs ..NOTHING MORE. If they happen to ALSO be "Eye Candy", just consider it a bonus! Although it should NOT be true that fact is that most people base a Personal Trainer's credibility on "looks" instead of knowledge and expertise. This can be - and often is - a BIG MISTAKE. In other words, if a female Personal Trainer happens to be Fitness Model, or if a male Personal Trainer has won a few local bodybuilding titles, they may STILL be as dumb as a doornail. Extremely fit or exceptionally attractive job-seekers are drawn to the Personal Training profession much like girls with flawless skin wanting to work the makeup counter at the mall, or guys with bulging biceps ending up working at the local supplement store. What they are really attempting to SELL is "You can look like me!" Sorry, we ALL wished it was that easy, it's NOT. I'm not even certain we can blame them. After all, we make it so easy for them to succeed solely on their body or looks; namely, with our own ignorance. You may feel compelled to ask, "Are you saying that someone who possesses bulging muscles, cannot ALSO have a brain, or a clue?" Of course I'm not, and of course they can. Many of my Personal Trainer friends actually do possess both. We call them "Lucky SOB's". However, most of them, if being truthful, would freely admit that having the perfectly balanced mesomorphic physique - the type that wins bodybuilding titles - has MORE to do with genetics, and LESS to do with anything they deserve credit for. Train hard? Of course, YOU MUST! However, if the genetic gods dealt you a pair of 2's instead of a Straight Flush - them's da breaks. TIP: Always interview any Personal Trainer you are considering hiring; credible ones will not mind at all. They should be able to easily explain their exercise philosophy and "why' it makes sense. They should be articulate in their command of basic exercise principles in a manner which oozes credibility. trust your gut; it's rarely wrong. A "qualified" Personal Trainer can be a tremendous asset in your quest to reach exercise goals. Just be sure, you're getting one.

Don't Follow This "Yellow Brick Road"

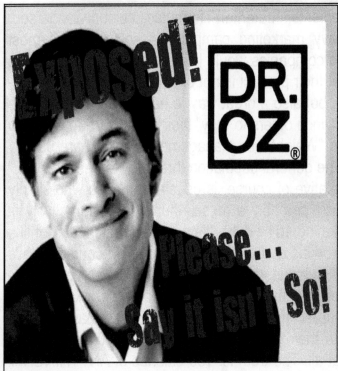

Yes, Dr. OZ is a "real" doctor. Many folks depend on him for his informed point of view on health topics. My opinion is that he often betrays that trust by increasingly and more often than not saying things "only" to help frauds SELL their BS. I have learned some neat stuff while occasionally watching his TV-show. HOWEVER, when he starts disguising "Infomercial" garbage as "real" unbiased educational information, he starts to lose me - and his credibility. Recently, the Dr. Oz Show had beachbody's Shawn T on as a guest. With this, I have no problem. Shawn's a swell guy and a great exercise instructor. If Shawn T was appearing to tell his story, be interviewed, or perhaps give factual exercise tips, that's fine. Instead, DR. OZ took part in an infomercial-type format. He touted ShawnT as having the "15-Min Miracle Workout" that helped "his" (DR. OZ's) family. That's an outright lie! DR. OZ has no business calling anything a "miracle" exercise prescription - he knows better. He further went on to say that ShawnT has "revolutionary-rules to burn fat all day". Again, the words "revolutionary", "secret", and "miracle" are usually associated with someone being full of crap, and again, the great DR. OZ knows better. Unfortunately, I do expect to be bombarded with beachbody Coach comments; So be it. I have many beachbody coach "friends" who are great people and knowledgeable exercise instructors. Many of us have even became "real" friend despite opposing stand on P90X. It's all good. In my opinion, DR.OZ (in this case) mislead and lied to his audience. In other words, it looks like he "sold-out". I guess you can decide for yourself? Here's the link if you're interested: http://www.youtube.com/watch?v=Cf8ny8Ww4Lc (Beachbody, ShawnT, and Dr. Oz are registered trademarks.)

Those "Magic" Weight-loss Shakes

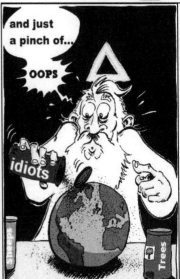

Exotic ingredients, "patented" formulas, celebrity-endorsed, etc. The heavy marketing campaign associated with most Shake-Selling companies would lead most unsuspecting folks to believe that their product is not only the holy-grail of weight-loss success, but also a great way to earn BIG $$ helping the company convince others to "buy" their own "Start-up Kit." Pah-lease! These "Weight-loss Management Shakes" are usually marketed to the general population through "Representatives." The representative of course, is usually someone who simply looks the part - probably a muscle-hunk or an attractively fit woman (Marketing 101 - duh). It's a perfect match, sort of like a pretty girl working at the cosmetic counter. Of course, what's being implied is that is you use the product you can be beautiful too. Most intelligent women have learned the hard way – it doesn't work that way. UNIQUE PATENTED FORMULA: Most up-scale Weight-loss Magic Shake Marketers follow a common recipe-makeup to create their own "unique-sounding" 100-or-so calorie drink - which is actually not so unique at all. The truth is: 100-calories of ANYTHING will qualify as a weight-loss meal - duh. Mostly ALL of these-type drinks will contain some exotic sounding "unique" ingredient, usually from lands far away, implying secret magical-powers that only the "natives" have known about for years. For example, one such drink contains something called Cha de Bugre - a Brazilian "slimming-herb" (yeah, right) It is also common for supplement companies to concoct a blend of different proteins in exact amounts, and then slap a "trademark" or "patented" label on it therefore creating an exclusive and unique magical blend. It is nothing more than a slick marketing trick. Shake Manufacturers usually add trace-amounts of an A-Z assortment of vitamins and minerals, mostly because it looks good on the ingredients-label. Getting the picture? "OUR OWN RESEARCH SAYS..." The last bit of trickery is the "Team" of Scientist or even a real doctor on-board to "verify" that cutting-edge science was used to create all these unique formulas. These schmucks are merely paid spokespersons. Yes, real doctors can be on-board as a means of supplementing their income. It can be VERY convincing. BOTTOM LINE: Exercise wisely, and learn how to eat REAL FOOD in healthy amounts.

"90-Day Challenges" Target the Clueless

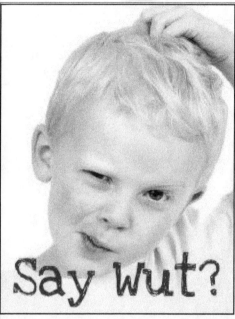

Say wut?

TV Infomercials and Local Gyms are Promoting Various Versions of The "90-Day Challenge". DON'T Get Burned By This 90-DAY Scam!

If You Read Between the Lines...Here's What They're REALLY Saying:

"Hey you, How would you like to transform your body in 90-Days and make a TON of CASH while doing it? Try our 90-Day Challenge. Each week simply buy our Meal Replacement Shakes, Energy-packs, Fat-burning Tabs, Meal-bars, and Detox-system Flush. This stuff really DOESN'T work, but don't worry 'cause we've created some really cool-sounding names for each product. We've even patented the stuff, which doesn't prove the stuff works, but it does sound really convincing even if you're NOT a MORON...but, we're hoping YOU ARE! We've even recruited pretty Fitness-Models and Awesome Bodybuilders to convince you that this is the "greatest product" they've ever used! The really, really cool thing is that if you get some of your friends to sell this stuff too, it will pay for the crap we want you to buy too! Our awesome company is really just one big lean n' mean, money-making family. We even go on Cruises to hold our Rah-Rah Meetings. Isn't this super-duper exciting? What are you waiting for? Order your first shipment today! We're giving away great prizes because we want to reward you for losing weight. You'll actually never win the grand prize, but you'll meet someone who really did, and they're really cool too! They'll get you so motivated you'll buy tons more of our stuff! If anybody with a real brain tries to say this stuff doesn't work, tell them that the 2011 Mr. All-Galaxy Winner, and the 2009 Miss Fluff n' Nutter Crown Winner both say our products kicks-ass! I actually lost 50-pounds in 3-days! Let me show you how..."

People fall for this nonsense every day...
Don't Be One.

Chapter 2

EATING
& WEIGHT-LOSS?
Ahhh... Now I Get It!

Will The Real "Diet Expert" Please Stand-Up?

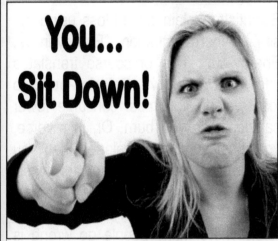

This is simple: In the United States, a **Registered Dietitian** is the accepted gold-standard for nutritional information. They are essentially "Diet Doctors". In-fact, a Registered Dietitian is who your Primary Care Physician consults with whenever dietary issues arise. They are the real diet experts. Look at these job-titles; they mean absolutely NOTHING:

"Diet Coach" "Nutritionist" "Herbalist"

"Diet Consultant" "Health Coach"

"Nutritional Expert" "Weight-Loss Guru"

Here's the point: Consumers should smarten-up, because the aforementioned "Job Titles" possess no accredited education pre-requisites, and have no legal validity what-so-ever. Anyone can legally give themselves one of these "fake" titles. A real Dietitian has to finish a Bachelor's degree in Nutrition and Dietetics or Graduate degree with the internship to be qualified. Registered Dietitians have met specific academic and experiential requirements set forth by each country's Dietetic Association Board universally. The credential RD (Registered Dietitian) is legally protected and a nationally recognized title and it can only be used by those whose are authorized by the particular country's Dietetic Association. Beware of "who" you receive your dietary and nutritional advice from.

The "Golden Rule" of Weight-Loss

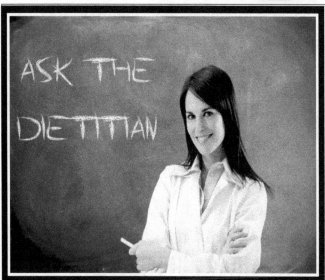

Scientists explain weight-loss using the simple energy-equation; "Energy-in vs. Energy-out". This of course translates into, **"Calories-in vs. Calories-out".** To lose weight, you must consume fewer calories than you burn. Or, in reverse, you must burn more calories than you consume. If you understand this basic fundamental of weight-loss, you understand nearly EVERYTHING that matters. Where many people go wrong is engaging in "fuzzy math". In other words, they believe - or are led to believe - that by introducing another factor into the simple energy-equation, it will make the weight-loss happen more quickly. Yes, I am talking about supplements, macro-ratios, low-carb, etc. The truth is, any reasonably healthy diet will work. Simply pick one and then stick to it. The default answer to every question regarding faster methods of weight-loss (i.e. special diet, unique exercise routines, energy supplements, fat-burners, metabolism boosters, etc.) is this: *Nothing supersedes the energy equation, "calories-in vs. calories-out", nor does anything make it irrelevant to weight-loss.* Most people get confused about "Calories". What they are, and how many you need to eat. A calorie is actually a unit of heat measurement. It measures the energy in food and beverages you consume. Everything we do relies on the energy that comes in the form of calories. The food we eat becomes the fuel that runs your body, even while you're sleeping your body is continuously burning calories. If this process stopped – you'd stop too - You're dead. It takes 3500 unused calories to produce one pound of body-fat. Your body is in a constant state of calories-in vs. calories-out. So, quite simply, when your body takes in more calories than it needs, it has NO choice but to store those extra calories as body-fat. So, How many calories per-day should you be eating? That depends on factors such as your current body-composition, activity level, age, etc. Use this formula: *Your Desired body-weight (the "weight" you're trying to reach) multiplied by twelve. For example; You weigh 187 lbs., but*

The "Golden Rule" of Weight-Loss

would like to weigh 145 lbs. Your math equation would look like this 145 X 12 = 1745 Calories per-day. This is a ball-park-figure. It allows you to select a logical starting point to your own calorie needs per-day. Also, DO NOT go below 1200 calories per day, regardless of what the "math" says. If nothing else, remember this: "A calorie is a calorie, period. This is so frequently misunderstood. Whether the calories you consume each day come from Protein, Carbohydrates, or Fats...THEY ARE ALL THE SAME. 3500 calories from vegetables will create the same pound of fat, as 3500 calories of Chocolate Fudge. Don't miss the point, yes, getting the majority of your daily calories from nutritious foods is the overall goal, but don't confuse this with being able to eat as much as you want just because you're eating "healthy", "low-fat", or "no-fat" food. Remember, calories differ "nutritionally", but NOT "calorically". Here's what REALLY matters when you choose your NEXT diet:

1– The Diet MUST Create a CALORIE DEFICIT. It doesn't really matter "What" you are eating daily; Good foods, Bad foods, or, a combination of both. If you are eating MORE calories than YOU are using, then yes, expect to get FATTER. Calories-in vs. calories-out is, and always will be, the Golden Rule of weight-loss. Nothing trumps it, or makes it not so.

2– The Diet MUST Be HEALTHY. Don't get me wrong - you actually CAN lose weight on an unhealthy diet. However, the longer you stay on such a diet, the more negative health issues you will (eventually) encounter. You simply CANNOT withhold nutrition from your body for very long - that's just stupid. The truth is, ANY reasonably healthy diet WILL work. Don't over-think things such as how many Carbs you are eating, the macro-nutrient ratio of your meals, or the difference between 3, 4, or 6 meals per day. Pick ANY sensible diet, and the, stick to it. TIP: The greatest weight-loss strategy ever, is "Portion Control". Remember, it's not WHAT we eat that gets us in trouble - it's HOW MUCH we eat. Too many people fall for gimmicky-diets because they are too lazy and too busy looking for a short cut. This is WHY Weight-loss is a billion dollar business. P.T. Barnum said, "There's a "Sucker" Born Every Minute!" He was right. If your NEXT diet strategy involves a delivery from Fed-EX, or a trip to the Supplement Store, you are probably headed for ANOTHER failed attempt at weight-loss. Smarten up.

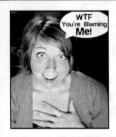

Here's The REAL Reason You May Be FAT

The Fitness and Weight-loss Industry is notorious for launching ad-campaigns which blames such things as a slow-metabolism, food additives, gluten, carbohydrate-sensitivity - blah-blah-blah - for the reason you are FAT. That's nonsense. Your real answer lies in honestly assessing your "Lifestyle". For the sake of this discussion, your lifestyle is something totally different than your income-level, the size of your home, or what kind of car you drive. Your lifestyle - as it pertains to how your body currently looks - is the total sum of ALL your **daily-behaviors** and **daily-habits**. They all have a dramatic impact on the way your naked-body looks in that full length mirror. This would include both your work-place and recreational activity-level. In other words, is your job, labor-intensive, or is it mostly sedentary in nature? The same can be asked regarding your spare-time. Do you workout at the gym or engage in physically demanding activities, or are you more of a couch-potato? Again, the answer is probably obvious as you study your reflection in the mirror. The other big lifestyle factor is your "eating-habits". You probably don't need much of an explanation here. The old adage "You are what you eat" , quite simply is true. It is important to understand that much more than genetics, how you have treated your body inside and out is what matters most. How much do you eat and how much do you move? - How many daily calories do you consume? What daily food choices are you making? Is your job a sedentary activity or does it involve manual labor? Do you exercise? If yes, how much and how often? If no, why not? Are you a busy-body, or do you look for ways to move less? Do you eat to fuel your body, or do you sometimes eat out of boredom, or as a stress-coping mechanism? Are you getting the picture? They all add up - These daily habits makeup your "lifestyle"...this is who you are...this is "why" you look the way you do...for better, or for worse. **The Good News:** Every one of your daily-habits and daily-behaviors can be altered, managed, or changed. Therefore, your body can change. This is the key to looking your best. By tweaking the way you eat, and when-and-how-often you move, you can dramatically impact the way your body looks. You DO NOT have to go on a "diet". You DO NOT have to spend hours exercising. Everything you need to know can be found between the front and back covers of this book. Starting here and now, take ownership of the problem. And then, make the appropriate lifestyle changes.

"Weight-Loss Resolutions" WHY They Fail

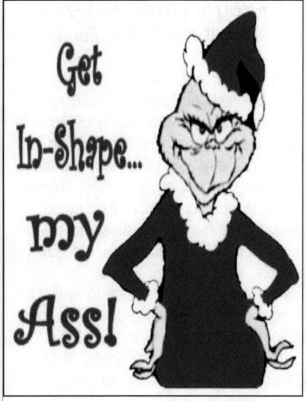

Are You REALLY Making Another Years New Year's Resolution to Lose Weight? If so, There are the two most common reasons they often fail.

Reason #1 - The "Status Quo Bias". You're probably saying, "Huh, what is that?" Real simple. It's a term behavioral scientist use. In a nutshell, we all have our own unique pattern of daily behaviors (our routines) that usually don't change much day to day. In the case of your "out-of-shape" body, it's your own eating and activity pattern that most likely got you into this - out of shape - mess in the first place. As you attempt to make beneficial lifestyle changes in your eating habits, like "portion control", or changes in your activity-level, like a new "exercise-regimen", predictably, your mind and body will resist. Again, it doesn't LIKE change. Fight back by knowing that reduced-calorie eating DOES occasionally suck, but, in time, your NEW behaviors will become your body's new "norm", and it'll get easier and easier. The NEW BODY you start seeing in your full length mirror will help too.

Reason #2 - The "PLAN" Itself. If this year's resolution to change your body has anything to do with "waiting for UPS" to deliver it, or a "trip to GNC" for a month's supply, or a new diet your idiotic co-workers are trying, oh brother, you're probably setting yourself up for another year's disappointment. This New Year's Resolution to lose weight or be more fit has EVERYTHING to do with "YOU" and your "PLAN". Use the information in this book to help you start making smart and sensible choices. It's really not that complicated.

"I'm IN-LOVE!" (with food that is)

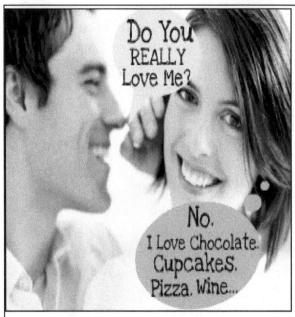

Are YOU in a DYSFUNCTIONAL RELATIONSHIP With Food?

Fact: Research suggests that 75% of the time we feel like "eating" something, it's for a reason other-than our body actually "needing it" for nourishment. Wow! In other words, only 25% of the time we eat is because our body actually needs nourishment. We eat for comfort, as a stress release, as a reaction to stress, to reward ourselves, out of boredom, etc. Often, people describe their reason for over-eating this way: "I just love to eat!" Our mind actually controls our eating frequency more than our stomach does. For many people, their "mind" is making poor decisions for our stomach. Ask yourself this question: Which do I love more: "Eating food?", or "Looking your best?" Here's the bad news: If your honest answer is truly, "eating food", ahead of "looking and feeling your best" then you will probably not maintain adherence to ANY fat-loss strategy. The great information found in this book, as informative and as simplified as it is, WILL NOT work on its own. "You" alone have to pull the trigger on adopting a new food mind-set. In other words, you might say you must change your "Dysfunctional relationship" with food. It's the largest part of the fat-loss puzzle. It is even MORE important than exercise. When people say "Oh she can eat whatever she wants, she works-out", they're WRONG. Think of it this way: A 130-pound woman, running a 26-mile marathon, would burn a total of (approx.) 2600 calories. If she rewarded herself (and she "would" deserve it) with a medium pepperoni pan-pizza, she would in-fact have just replace ALL the calories burned in running the marathon. Again, exercise will NEVER cancel-out stuffing your face. **The cliché may need to change. Instead of saying, "We Are WHAT We Eat"....It should read: "We Are HOW MUCH We Eat".**

Frosting, Bacon, or Ice Cream Has NEVER Made Anybody FAT!

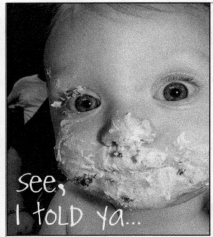

see, I told ya...

Here's something EVERY "Dieter" should realize, and EVERY Fitness Professional should be passing along to their "Weight-loss" Clients. Many people don't seem to understand is that "Food" is NOT fattening; "Excessive Calories" IS fattening! You may be saying, "Isn't that the same thing?" No, not really. It's more the PORTION SIZES of any food that gets us in trouble, not the particular TYPE of food. For example, one-half stick of butter is actually LESS fattening than - say - a large bowl of oatmeal and raisins. How can this be true? It's because the butter equals 400-calories, yet the large cereal-bowl of oatmeal and raisins equals approximately 600-calories. In other words, Butter and Bacon are two foods that are certainly viewed by most of us as "fattening". However, one Tablespoon of butter has only 100-calories; the same for a small strip of bacon; about 100-calories. NOBODY CAN GET FAT ON 100-CALORIES OF ANYTHING. However, if you load-up on butter too often, your overall calorie-intake will then become excessive, and as a result, so will the amount of fat being deposited on your ass, thighs, and belly. The RULE remains true; If you eat too much low-fat yogurt, oatmeal, or raisins, the calories begin to add, and so do the pounds. Again, it's the "AMOUNTS of FOODS" that gets us in trouble, NOT a particular food. Make sense? The "amount" of food you eat, or more specifically, the number of "calories" you eat over the course of a days, weeks, and months. This is what results in weight-loss, or weight-gain, not the fact that you ate a hot-fudge sundae today. That said, common sense dictates that we should ALWAYS strive to eat primarily healthy foods. However, it's crazy to think that you can't mix in "high-fat" or "sugary" treats here n' there. Or, as they say: "Everything in Moderation". I cringe when people say "I'm cutting out butter, cream, and all desserts...they're ALL so fattening!" I realize that they probably don't "get it", and as a result, they needlessly over-deprive themselves, and make their own weight-loss strategy one that's harder to stick-to. **BOTTOM-LINE: Common sense and an occasional strip of bacon or bowl of ice cream here n' there will allow ANY diet to be more bearable, and therefore - in the long run - more successful.**

"CARBS" Do NOT Make You FAT!

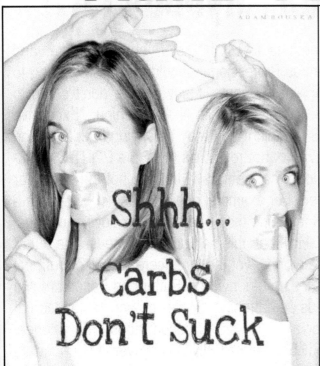

I Once Heard a TV "Diet Expert" Make the Following Statement:

Quote: *"Because, Carbohydrates produce a release of Insulin into the bloodstream, and since Insulin is a "fat storage" hormone, if you limit your carbs, no insulin can be released, and therefore, no fat storage can occur."* OH REALLY? Before you say "OMG! Carbs really do make me fat!", trust me, this "Expert" is NO expert. Like many myths, this one too, is born out of shreds of truth and twisted logic. The main reason for our insulin fear is the common belief that sugary foods cause insulin to be released into the bloodstream, and since Insulin is commonly referred to as a "fat storage" hormone, we therefore believe that Insulin is capable of turning a few Hershey's Kisses or a bagel into instant body-fat. That's just nonsense. First of all, we need to understand is that Insulin is a "good thing" - just ask any Type-1 Diabetic who's body can't produce enough on its own. The truth is, a rise in blood-sugar comes from nearly "anything" we eat, even foods that are low on the glycemic index charts, if they're eaten in a large quantity. **KNOW THIS:** If you are prone to hyper-fluctuating blood-sugar levels, the two main things you NEED to avoid are LARGE MEALS and foods which are made-up of CARBS entirely. The reason of course, is that a hyper insulin-response results from BOTH the "quantity" of the food eaten, and how "quickly" certain foods break down when digested, i.e. simple sugars and high glycemic foods. **TIP: You can ACTUALLY control the insulin response from pure carbs and sugars, in two different ways: 1 - Control the PORTION SIZE of foods you eat** (The benefit is obvious...the more calories you consume in a single sitting, the more insulin response there will be – even if it's a low-carb food). **2 - A Trick: Combine FAT or FIBER with hi-sugar foods.** (This actually SLOWS-DOWN the rate of digestion of any food, and therefore, the rate at

"CARBS" Do NOT Make You FAT!

which it gushes into your bloodstream). **Translation:** That plain baked potato, which may cause a quick blood sugar response, suddenly slows down with pat of butter or reasonable dollop of sour cream added to it. I'll bet you never thought you'd hear someone say that butter or sour cream can be a "good thing". By knowing the relationship between Insulin, blood sugar, carbs, fiber, and fat, it may allow you to enjoy ANY food in moderation, even dreaded Carbs. The best eating strategy is, and always will be, POR-TION CONTROL. Find ways to fit goodies n' treats into a healthy diet. Take-away: Carbs DO NOT make you FAT - Too MANY Carbs DO (Just like any other calorie). **Important Side Note:** You may hear and read internet blogs that attempt to bring the relationship between **"Carbs"** and **"Type 2 Diabetes"** into their argument. It tends to usually be Paleo or Atkin's Diet advocates. Unfortunately, although Low-Carb Diets have been effective for some people, and yes, when a person's diagnosed with Type-2 Diabetes, a lower-carb eating strategy will probably be recommended by your (Registered) Dietitian. That said, this type of eating is NOT embraced as the diet for the masses or average person. In the US, Registered Dietitians are STILL the Gold-Standard for nutritional expertise. Their conscientious is STILL that weight-loss has mostly to do with an overall calorie-deficit. Yup, **"Calories-In vs. Calories-Out" is the Golden Rule.** In case you don't really understand what Type-2 Diabetes actually is, or how you'd get it, here's a briefer than it should be explanation. T2D, as it is often referred to, develops when the body becomes resistant to insulin or when the pancreas stops producing enough insulin. The truth is, the medical community still does not totally understand it, or exactly why this happens. That said, it "is" widely believe within credible science circles that **being over-weight and and/or inactive** do seem to be contributing factors. Too many genetic variables or unknowns I suspect. The important thing is that when considering any dietary strategy, you can actually argue for or against ANY reasonably healthy diet. In other words, they ALL work. Macronutrient ratios and such is more often than not merely "semantics" for marketing purposes (hawking a product)...or simply a matter of splitting hairs between knowledgeable individuals who are actually more in-agreement than not about what's really important; which is, having a basic understanding of weight-loss science. Always be guided by credible nutritional science, a good dose of common sense, and your own (dietary) trials n' errors to find what works best for "you." This will ALWAYS be the best DIET advice ever.

Protein or Carbs?
The Good-Guy/Bad-Guy Carousel

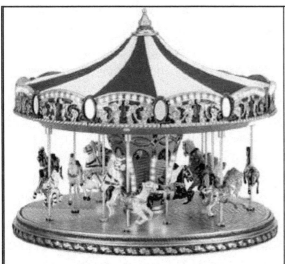

PROTEIN & CARBS
The Good-Guy - Bad-Guy
Carousel.

Over decades I have seen the cyclical rotation of Protein, Carbohydrates, and Fat, each having their turn being viewed as a dietary "Bad Guy". In the 70's Carbs were the Food Superstar. Carbs, carbs, carbs, was the battle cry of every coach and athlete. Fast-forward to today, suddenly Carbs are the villain. And, who the hell ever thought Fat would sprint to the front of the pack in one of today's most diets - The Atkins Diet. **This is not intended to be a lesson on Nutrition.** I am assuming everybody "gets" that protein is a meat, dairy, nuts, and legumes-type food, and that Carbohydrates are fruits, vegetables, sugars, sweets, and grain products (breads-pasta-etc.). I simply want to clear up some common misconceptions and provide an "in-a-nutshell" overview of the two. **Here's the scoop on Protein & Carbs...**

PROTEIN
(The Building Blocks of Our Body)

How much should I eat? 35% - 45% of your overall daily calorie intake. Experts (the real ones) differ in their recommendation, yet most do agree on a number within this range. So don't micro-manage your exact %. Try to stay within this range - give or take - and you'll be okay. **More Protein means Bigger Muscles, right? NO!** This myth has been around since man first realized he "had" Muscles. Because the body uses dietary protein to make muscle, then more protein must mean more muscle, right?

Protein or Carbs?
The Good-Guy/Bad-Guy Carousel

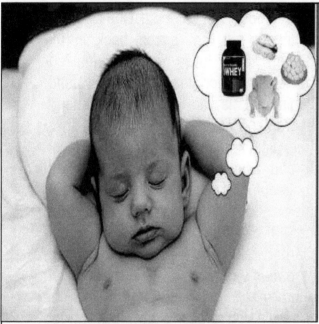

Wrong. More protein - beyond your needs - simply means more calories - period.

CARBOHYDRATES (Carbs)
(The Energy that Fuels Our Body)

How Many Carbs? 50% - 60% of your overall daily calorie intake. Again, most experts (real ones) differ in their recommendation. Again, most do agree on number within this range. So don't micro-manage your exact %. Just try to stay within this range - give or take - and you'll be okay...no biggie. **Carbs will make me fat? NO!** Too many carbohydrates in the form of gluttony will make you fat, but not any more than too much protein, or too much fat. Extra calories makes you fat! It doesn't matter which kind. A calorie, is a calorie - period. **Carbs provide super energy, right?** Energy, yes! Super energy, not quite. The body takes what it needs from dietary carbohydrates, and stores the rest as fat. The "super energy" claims that come from Energy-Drinks are misleading. They're simply sugar-drinks in expensive packaging...don't be fooled.

Protein and Carbs are both important in any healthy diet, but neither have the magical ability to build huge muscles, or, give you super-energy.

Good FAT - Bad FAT
The Good, the Bad, & the Ugly

Servings per Container about 12 about 2 servings (cups) per bag 6 bags per container	
Amount Per Serving	**As Packaged**
Calories	190
Calories from Fat	0
	% Daily Value*
Total Fat 0g	**0%**
Saturated Fat 0g	**0%**
Trans Fat 0g	
Cholesterol 0mg	**0%**
Sodium 0mg	0%

The Good: Fat is good! Don't get too excited... put that bacon back in the fridge! Dietary fat is a vital nutrient our bodies need for health and daily functioning. It is an outstanding energy source and promotes healthy skin, shiny hair, vitamin-absorption, and regulation of bodily functions. Fat is also essential to keeping you feeling full in between meals. So far, so good! **The Bad:** Fat has 9 calories per-gram. Protein and Carbohydrates have 4 calories per-gram each. Although a calorie is a calorie, too many "fatty-food" choices will usually mean too many calories, which in-turn means calories stored as fat. **The Ugly:** Although fat is both good and bad, if you're eating too much fat, too often - everybody will know because it'll end up on your belly, butt, and thighs. **There are different types of fat in the foods we eat. This is all you have to remember: Poly and Mono-unsaturated fats** = GOOD! **Saturated -fats** = NOT SO GOOD! **Trans-fats** = VERY BAD **Poly-unsaturated fats** and **Mono-unsaturated fats** are both found in foods like nuts, certain fish varieties, olive oil, and for-that-matter, cooking oils that are vegetable in origin (Corn, Safflower, Soybean, Canola, Etc.). These types of fat can lower your risk for certain diseases, especially heart disease. **Saturated fats** are found mainly in full-fat dairy foods, meats, certain oils, most bakery products, etc. These types of fat can increase the risk for certain diseases, especially heart disease. **The key is to substitute good fats for bad fats whenever you can. While we're on the subject, I may as well give you a rundown on these two trouble-makers: Trans-fat and Cholesterol. Trans-fat** is vegetable oil (good fat) that has been transformed into bad fat by a process

Good FAT - Bad FAT
The Good, the Bad, & the Ugly

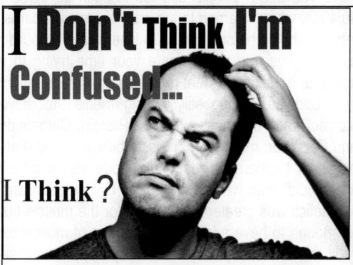

I Don't Think I'm Confused...

I Think?

called, "Hydrogenation". Pre-packaged baked goods, donuts, cup-cakes, and other com-mercially prepared foods are usually major sources of trans fats. Why do they do this? It has to do with shelf-life, texture-of-food, etc. Bot-tom line: Whenever pos-sible, don't eat it. **Cho-lesterol:** Again, good news-bad news. Cholesterol is not actually a fat, but a waxy fat-like substance. It is produced in the body naturally. The body uses it for GOOD things. However, in excess it can lead to heart problems. Like sat-urated fat, it is found in animal foods such as beef and shellfish. A high level of cholesterol in the blood is a major risk factor for coronary heart-disease, and also increases the risk of stroke. 300 mg of cholesterol daily is what the experts (the real ones) generally agree on. **The important thing to know about Cholesterol is that high blood-levels are actually more of a he-redity issue, than a dietary one. Generally speaking, heart disease tends to run in families. Therefore, take a good look at your family tree, and then, live your life accordingly.**

Important Note: There are actually some credible studies lately that show that "saturated fats" may not be as harmful as once thought. That said, until it becomes conclusive, it's still a good idea to careful when consuming them. The bulk of the evidence to-date, still says they're "not so good."

Don't Over-Think "Macro-Nutrient Ratios"

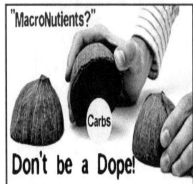

"MacroNutients?"

Carbs

Don't be a Dope!

Have you heard people use terms such as 60/30/10 or 40/40/20 when referring to the ratio of proteins, carbs, and fats we should be consuming to lose weight or build more muscle. Trust me, don't waste your time trying to make sense of it. Macro-nutrient ratios is latest craze among my gym buddies. Supposedly, eating meals that have the "correct" ratio of macro-nutrients (Protein, Carbohydrates, and Fats) can make both "muscle-building" and "Fat-loss" magically happen. Oh really? Anybody who has tried this macro tweaking diet strategy and "did" lose weight, did so for ONE reason and one reason alone; an overall calorie-deficit was created, period. As for the muscle-building nonsense, if you are fortunate enough to have added a few pounds of muscle to your body, you should be giving credit to the intensity and consistency of your exercise program, and NOT a magical ratio of protein intake. Remember, a calorie, is a calorie, is a calorie. It doesn't matter the source of the food. Even "healthy" foods, if eaten in excess amounts will soon cause anyone to get fatter. On the other hand, eating a diet consisting of only junk-food, if eaten in amounts that result in an over-all calorie deficit, will make you shed fat. It's really a simple energy balance equation, no matter WHAT the Low-Carb advocates say. In a perfect world, yeah, I guess if every meal we ate was perfectly balanced that would be a good thing. But, a "magical" thing, no. In the over-all scheme of things, the macro-ratio percentages of your meals are really not that important. Your body really doesn't care much about the percentage of protein, carbs, and fat each meal contains (unless of course there is a medical-issue in-play). All that's important to your body is that over the course of the day, or days, it's getting enough of each to satisfy its needs for health, growth, and repair. Therefore, in magazine articles or eating blogs, when you see macro-nutrient combination-numbers such as, 40/40/20, or 50/40/10, or even 40/20/40. What do they mean? The short answer is, NOT ENOUGH TO GET OVERLY CONCERNED ABOUT. Our eating-habits should ALWAYS be guided by credible nutritional-science, logic, common-sense, and your own experiences. Nobody with a qualified brain would ever argue against this advice.

"Vitamins"
Let's NOT Get Carried Away

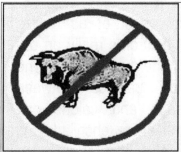

Are "Vitamins" Essential? Yes ...But Let's NOT Get Carried Away. Vitamins are known as "micro-nutrients" for a reason. Our bodies need them in only teenie-weenie amount to be effective at what they do; namely work in-concert with food to perform little tasks in our bodies that keep us healthy. Without turning this into a lesson on "Nutrition", which should only come from a Registered Dietician, and NOT some dip-shit "Diet Counselor", "Food Coach", or other Moron possessing a title that has no legal-meaning or accreditation whatsoever. To many people are mistakenly gobbling-up mouthfuls of vitamins for the "wrong" reasons. My personal beef is that people mistakenly think that vitamins possess properties and abilities to do things in our bodies that are just NOT true. Mostly because some Gym-Brainiac is, as usual, spewing misinformation or selling stuff that can't possibly do what's being promised. I wanted to share a few of my favorite vitamin and mineral myths and misconceptions regarding "energy" and "fat-burning". **MYTH: B-Vitamins give You "Energy".** Wrong! Food gives us energy, NOT vitamins. This common misconception is (mostly) believed because "B-vitamins" do act as a catalyst in the process of releasing energy from the carbohydrates we eat. Supplements like "5-Hour Energy" like to tout that their product contains Vitamin B-6. It does. However, it does absolutely nothing for you as far providing "energy". **MYTH: "Lecithin" Dissolves Fat in Your Body**. Nope! This one's easy; Lecithin is a nutrient compound that is used as an "emulsifier" in foods. Because of these properties, it's easy to see how some Supplement makers convince us to take the leap that it can emulsify or "melt" the fat in our bodies. Nonsense! **MYTH: Chromium Picolinate Helps You Burn More Fat.** Wrong again! Chromium is a mineral that performs numerous functions in the body, including glucose and fat metabolism, and helping insulin to work efficiently in our bodies. Bodybuilders often take this supplement to "get ripped". Truth is - all they're "getting" is ripped-off! A common-practice used by supplement makers is to convince us the just because - say - "Nutrient XYZ" is involved in a certain process in our bodies, taking more Nutrient XYZ will super-charge that process. Of course we often believe it because the shreds of truth that make-up these claims seem at least plausible. More often than not - it's BS.

The Easiest DIET You've Never Tried

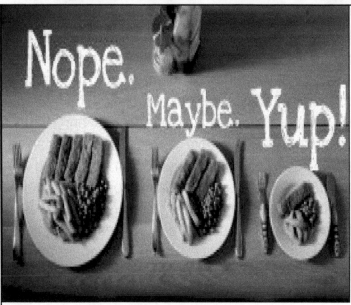

By now most of us realize weight-control is really an on-going energy-equation. The on-going balance between calories-in and calories-out. It's the entire enchilada. All you need to do to start seeing your body-fat melt away is tip the energy-equation scale in your favor, by consuming fewer-calories. You can NOT become lean by exercising alone. Exercise will never cancel out, stuffing your face. The real answer? "Portion Control". Don't be fooled by its simplicity. It's a powerful and effective strategy, when done correctly. This is manly true because Portion Control is the least restrictive form of eating. It's hard to stick to any diet that says you can only eat from a small group of food selections, or that "fat" or "carbs" are a no-no. When your family eats lasagna - now you can too. Portion control and a little common sense will allow you to eat ANYTHING you want. You get to eat the foods you always eat, yet by cutting the portion by - say - 50% - and presto! Instant calorie reduction. Instant fat-loss. **Tips:** Never fill a large dinner-plate and then say "I'll just eat half. It NEVER works. Also, when dining in restaurants, ask for a "to-go" container at the same time you order your meal. When served, immediately put half of the meal into the container. It will be another meal, at another time. Here's a method that I've seen work for many: Buy yourself a few really fancy dessert plates. They're about 5-6 inches in diameter. Each time you eat a meal, serve it to yourself on these plates. It will naturally keep the portion-size down, yet have the appearance of a "full-plate." Breakfast cereals can be eaten out of smaller bowls or coffee-mugs, and foods like creamy soups and ice cream are eaten out of tea-cups. Are you getting the picture? Give it a try.

If You MUST Choose a Popular Diet Here's That 3 Can't Miss

Heading into 2014, the U.S News & World Report assembled a panel of health experts who evaluated 2014's popular diets, and then ranked them according to healthiness and effectiveness. To be top-rated, a diet had to be relatively easy to follow, nutritious, safe and effective for weight loss and against diabetes and heart disease. The government-endorsed Dietary Approaches to Stop Hypertension (DASH) snagged the top spot. Here are there top-3 as reported in the AP.

No. 1: The DASH Diet. DASH was developed to fight high blood pressure, not as an all-purpose diet. But it certainly looked like an all-star to our panel of experts, who gave it high marks for its nutritional completeness, safety, ability to prevent or control diabetes, and role in supporting heart health. Though obscure, it beat out a field full of better-known diets. **The claim:** A healthy eating pattern is key to deflating high blood pressure—and it may not hurt your waistline, either. **The theory:** Nutrients like potassium, calcium, protein, and fiber are crucial to fending off or fighting high blood pressure. You don't have to track each one, though. Just emphasize the foods you've always been told to eat (fruits, veggies, whole grains, lean protein, and low-fat dairy), while shunning those we've grown to love (calorie- and fat-laden sweets and red meat). Top it all off by cutting back on salt, and ta-dah!

No. 2: The TLC Diet. Therapeutic Lifestyle Changes, or TLC, is a very solid diet plan created by the National Institutes of Health. It has no major weaknesses, and it's particularly good at promoting cardiovascular health. One expert described it as a "very healthful, complete, safe diet." But it requires a "do-it-yourself" approach, in contrast to the hand-holding provided by some commercial diets. **The claim:** You'll lower your "bad" LDL cholesterol by 8 to 10 percent in six weeks. **The theory:** Created by the National Institutes of Health's National Cholesterol Education Program, the Therapeutic Lifestyle Changes Diet (TLC) is endorsed by the American Heart Association as a heart-healthy regimen that can reduce the risk of cardiovascular disease. The key is cutting back sharply on fat, particularly saturated fat. Saturated fat (think fatty meat, whole-milk dairy, and fried foods) bumps up bad cholesterol, which increases the risk of heart attack and stroke. That, along with strictly limiting daily dietary cholesterol intake and getting more fiber, can help people manage high cholesterol, often without medication.

No. 3 (tie): Mayo Clinic. This is the Mayo Clinic's take on how to make healthy eating a lifelong habit. It earned especially high ratings from our experts for its nutrition and safety and as a tool against diabetes. Experts found it moderately effective for weight loss. **The claim:** You'll shed 6 to 10 pounds in two weeks and continue losing 1 to 2 pounds weekly until you've hit your goal weight **The theory:** You recalibrate your eating habits, breaking bad ones and replacing them with good ones with the help of the Mayo Clinic's unique food pyramid. The pyramid emphasizes fruits, veggies, and whole grains. In general, these foods have low energy density, meaning you can eat more but take in fewer calories. Think of it this way: For about the same amount of calories you could have a quarter of a Snicker's bar or about two cups of broccoli. **Note: The Mediterranean Diet and The Weight Watchers Diet tied for 3rd. More information on either diet can be easily found in a Google search.**

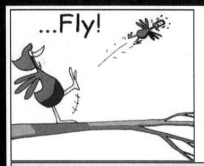

...Fly!

The 10-Commandments of "Tough-Love" Weight-Loss

#1 - Pah-Lease - Another Excuse? Just Do It!

Of ALL your past attempts to lose weight, how many times did you truly and totally commit to succeeding? Write this date on your calendar. Make it a big deal. Challenge yourself to not give-in when it becomes difficult; and more importantly, to get right back on track when or if you (occasionally) falter.

#2 - Reduced-Calorie Eating Can Sometimes Be Frustrating. Do It Anyway.

The attitude YOU bring to this plan is EVERYTHING! Don't complain to others that you "hate" having to eat this way. Instead, speak glowingly and confidently about your weight-loss plan. Perhaps use self-talk positive affirmations. Your body responds to your thoughts, and your thoughts create your reality. Remind yourself that you "love" this new "you". Remind yourself how great you feel, and how much greater you are becoming.

#3 - "How Many Calories Should You Eat?" (A Guide For the CLUELESS)

Multiply Your "Goal Weight" by 12. This will provide you with a ballpark figure of how many calories you need to consume daily to reach your target weight. For example, if you currently weigh 185 lbs., and are trying to reduce your weight down to a healthier - say - 140 lbs., you would then multiply 140 X 12. The total is 1680 calories daily...pretty simple. When you take-in this many calories you'll see change almost immediately. One important thing to remember is that you should never go below 1200 calories per day, no matter what the math says.

#4 - Get Tough With Your Non-Supporters

Amidst all the positives, the last thing you need is somebody dragging you down with negative thoughts and comments. It is crucial that the people closest to you; your spouse, friends, co-workers, etc., become a positive and supportive force. Have a heart-to-heart chat with any and all of these people. If they are simply hell-bent on dragging you down; re-think the relationship. Just sayin'.

#5 - This Time, Nutritional Density DOES Count.

I know you are used to me saying a "Calorie is a Calorie", or that you can get just as fat on 3500 calories of apples, as 3500 calories of bacon fat. It's still true. However, because you only have a limited number of daily-calories to nourish your body adequately, it becomes important that your food selections be from mostly healthy-foods. Plenty of fruit, vegetables, whole-grains, lean cuts of meat, etc. On occasions, when you want to enjoy - say - lasagna with your family, that's fine. You could then use a portion-control strategy. I wrote a great "Portion Control" post right here on my Facebook page Find it. Read it.

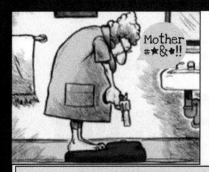

The 10-Commandments of "Tough-Love" Weight-Loss

#6 - For 3 STRAIGHT DAYS, Write Down Everything You Eat.

Nobody wants to live their life writing down everything they eat, I agree. That said, it is a great success tool for the first week of your new eating, mostly because it makes you conscious of everything you're putting in your mouth, and you are less likely to grab a nibble of this and just a taste of that if you have to write it down. Do not skip this step, it is such a powerful eating deterrent - you'll see.

#7 - DO NOT Exceed 500 Calories per Meal.

This is important for a couple reasons. First, meals much bigger than this will use up a bigger than necessary amount of your daily calorie allowance. In other words, you don't want to eat most of your daily allotment of calories in just one meal. Secondly, these smaller-type meals will help keep your blood-sugar stable, therefore helping control excessive blood-sugar fluctuations, which can lead to binging eating.

#8 - DO NOT Wait More than 6 Hours to Eat Your Next Meal.

Again, this has to do with keeping your blood-sugar stabilized and not setting yourself up for binge-eating. Simple, but important, because it is so easy to get caught in the "I'm not going to eat" trap. It ALWAYS Fails!

#9 - Are You Getting Hungry Again Within 3-hours of Eating?

If yes, it may be an emotional-eating issue, i.e., boredom, stress, etc. studies have shown that 75% of the time we reach for something to eat, it's for reasons other than our body actually needing nourishment. If you do not suspect that emotional eating is the culprit, try eating a higher amount of protein, fat, or fiber as part of your meals. This will help slow the absorption-rate of foods through your digestive-system and into your blood-stream, keeping you fuller, longer.

#10 - DO NOT Exercise Too Much (Say Wut?)

Nothing screws-up a diet more than over-exercising. It will put you in a rundown state which very often leads to lack of motivation, or even binge-eating. There is no need to plod-along on the treadmill 7-days/week for an hour or more, or to attend high impact exercise classes every day, or even multiple times per day. That's just crazy. I would rather see you doing strength-training 3-times per week. If you do decide to go strictly cardio, such as treadmill, elliptical, power-walking, or even running - limit it to no more than 3 times per week - which is plenty if done correctly. Think of going harder, rather than further. In other words, 20-minutes of interval-type cardio is far superior to constantly attempting to exercise longer. The fat-burning effect is greater with shorter, more intense cardio sessions.

Putting It ALL Together: What Should YOUR Plan Be?

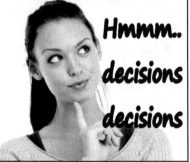

Hmmm.. decisions decisions

Think about this: You know "you" better than anyone else ever will. Based on what you've learned in this book, you should be able to select the lifestyle changes that are most likely to stick, and be successful for YOU. Will your success depend on a few minor lifestyle adjustments? Do you begin a new Exercise-regimen? Or, do you need to make changes in your current workout - which you may soon realize - doesn't make much sense. Will you make changes by simply "moving more" in the course of your daily-routine? Can you find ways to carve 500-calories-a-day out your eating-habits without missing them? Will your success come from much-needed portion-control? Will you STOP listening to the "Infomercial-Experts", now that you have a closet full of gadgets and videos that are useless? "What" will YOU decide to do? It's time to "personalizing" your strategy. The one rule that applies to everybody - yes, even you, is that the "only" way you are going to lose fat and change your body's appearance is to manage the balance between the calories you consume (eat), and the calories you expend (or burn). It really is this simple. You must make a conscious effort to move more (calories-out), and consume-less (calories-in). This weight-loss law will NEVER change. Begin at the beginning. As we've already discussed, it all begins with "you" making the needed changes in your own lifestyle. And then, have the motivational-fortitude and discipline to stick with it. You'll probably need to eat between 1500 and 3500 calories per-day, depending on your goal-weight. You don't have to over-think it - always attempt to eat an overall balance of protein, carbohydrates, and fats. They're all "good" - and they're all "bad"...it's how you use them that counts Too much of any equals extra pounds of fat. Yes, you probably should adopt some form of exercise regimen, even if it's simply "moving more" in your daily routine. Between your new eating habits and an increased activity-level, you should be seeking to create a daily 500 to 1000 calorie deficit. At a rate of just 500 per day, you will lose a pound of body-fat every seven days. It's actually not that difficult to lose 1-3 pounds per week, but it does take commitment to a plan. "Your" plan. *Don't Forget: To determine your (ballpark) daily caloric needs, multiply your goal-weight by 12 (Example: Goal-weight is 135 lbs. x 12 = 1620 calories/day). Make slight adjustments based on on-going results.*

Chapter 3

"EXERCISE RESULTS" Ahhh . . . Now I Get It!

Everything You THINK You Know About EXERCISE, is (Probably) Wrong!

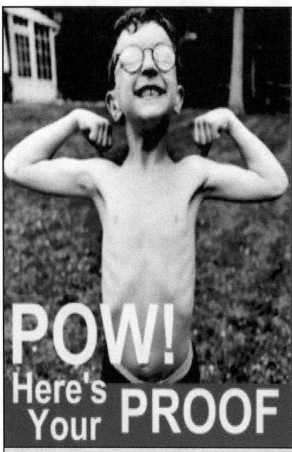

POW! Here's Your PROOF

The problem with too many exercise programs is that - quite frankly - they don't make sense. That's "if" you are expecting either to make changes in the way your body looks or to improve your muscular strength. Too much of what goes on in gyms and exercise classes everywhere is born out of myths, folklore, and workout fads. The "cause and effect" of exercise is something that too few exercise enthusiast truly understand. Instead, we continuously select the wrong exercises for the results we are then expecting to happen The most puzzling phenomenon in many instances is that although no results are achieved, people will STILL resist change. Myths and BS become so acceptable as fact, that even "no results" will not persuade some people to change. Incredible, isn't it. Everything in the upcoming pages regarding exercise is evidence-based or scientifically accurate. Don't be surprised if on more than one occasion, you find yourself saying, *"no way is that true!"* Well, *according to credible eating and exercise science, it is.*

So, Which is it... Who's Right?

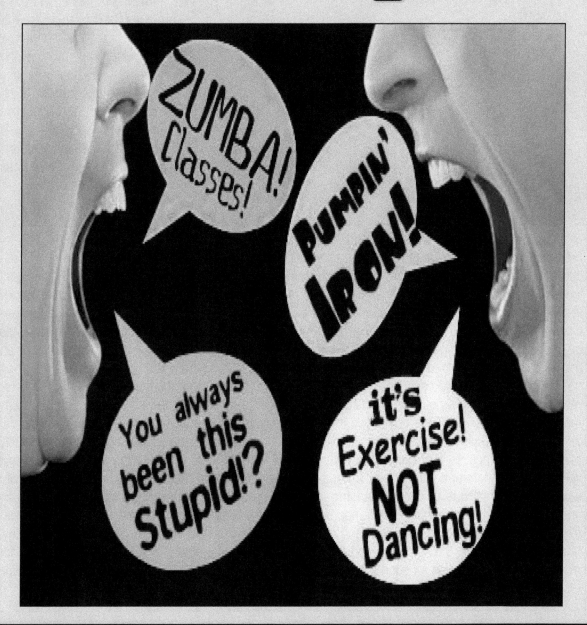

Are YOU Getting YOUR Best "Exercise Results?"

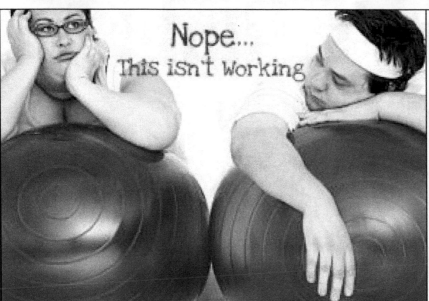

Exercise is meant to accomplish one-of-two things: **1 - Increase Our Muscular -Strength. 2 - Increase Our Cardiovascular Fitness.** I realize that a few readers may be thinking "Not me, my goal is to lose fat!" Fat-loss can be a direct result of productive exercise, but fat-loss is NOT a "type" of exercise. Remember, exercise can ONLY be productive "if" and "when" you make challenges to your body's current capacity to perform mechanical work. In other words, whether you're a bodybuilder trying to increase muscle-mass, an athlete trying to run a faster 400 meter race, or the average Joe trying to become more fit; You will not realize "any" improvements in your muscle-growth, your ability to run-faster longer, or become more fit in-general until you push your limits. It is only then that an "adaptive-response" takes place within your muscles, or cardiovascular-system. The adaptive response to exercise is what you should be shooting for whenever you exercise - that's if a change in your appearance or performance is your goal. Every time we exercise, workout, or train intensely enough to trigger an adaptive-response, our body then need 48-72 hours of rest to recuperate and get stronger. Whether-or-not there is an adaptive response to our exercise efforts has to do with whether-or-not the exercise reached the minimum amount of "intensity" to cause such a response - and I don't mean jackin' up as much weight as you can for a rep-or-two in the weight room, or jumping around in a ZUMBA class for an hour. Most people hinder their own ability to make progress in there exercise efforts by being guilty of one-or-two things: **1 - Not exercising with enough "intensity" to produce the adaptive-response needed to facilitate new strength or fitness-levels. 2 - Not being able to adequately recover from exercise-sessions due to over-exercising (e.g., too many sets or too much cardio).** My own personal pet-peeve is the aspiring muscle-heads who perform set-after-set and waste hours of time over-training in an obsession to get bigger and stronger. Or, women attending exercise classes everyday, becomes run-down in the process, and then quits exercise altogether. The Best exercise advice for most people is to exercise for shorter periods of time - but exercise harder. That of course is if getting the "best results" in the shortest amount of time is your goal is your goal.

"I Exercise But My Body NEVER Changes" Here's the Reason Why...

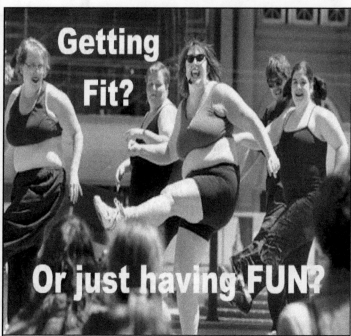

Getting Fit?

Or just having FUN?

It's so frustrating when I see people attending exercise classes like ZUMBA, Power Yoga, or Brazilian-Butt Classes 3-times per-week, who believe that it's going to change the way their body looks. It's NOT. The same goes for all those ladies jumping around - three-times per week - in ANY dance-type exercise class, and believing it's going to sculpt their arms, legs, and butt. It's NOT. Why? Because it Can't. Until you understand the CAUSE and EFFECT of EXERCISE, you may be wasting your time engaged in an exercise program that will NEVER do what you want it to do. That's IF your goal is weight-loss, or a firm sculpted body, which is according to the women I speak with, the #1 goal of MOST women.

THIS IS IMPORTANT: When people who take these-type classes say, "Yeah, but it worked for me - it changed my body", I always reply, "No, your DIET changed your body - your exercise classes were simply a fun activity you engage in 3 times per week". Rarely do I see FAT bodies - who regularly engage in Exercise Classes - change. Too many people (women mostly) believe that if they engage in an exercise class 3-4 times per, they are then doing their part to drop pounds. They are not. Aerobic exercise (per session) burns way fewer calories than many believe. "Torch up to 1000 calories in my class", is something Instructors are used to saying. Sorry, it's a lie. Exercise will NEVER cancel-out stuffing your face. REMEMBER: The EXERCISE PROGRAM you choose to engage in on a regular basis can ONLY DO what it is capable of doing, and it can NEVER do what it is NOT capable of doing." In other words, Zumba, Power Yoga, Les Mills Videos, Cardio-Pump Classes, Boot Camps, etc., may in fact be "fun", and yes, that does have some value, but because these-type exercise programs can NOT be progressively more intense by-nature, and because it is impossible to measure the amount of (if any) progressive over-loading of the musculature, these become poor exercise choices, IF, "measurable results" is your goal. VALID COUNTERPOINT: Look, I'll admit, if ZUMBA or Brazilian Butt Lift gets you motivated to exercise; so be it. It's great that you are doing "something". Besides, it may actually be the gateway to other exercise programs that can be more productive, such as high-intensity strength training, which by the way, is STILL the most scientifically-supported type of exercise to "CHANGE the WAY YOUR BODY LOOKS". Decide for yourself, is it time to CHANGE your exercise strategy?

Why Most Exercise Classes Are Filled with FAT People

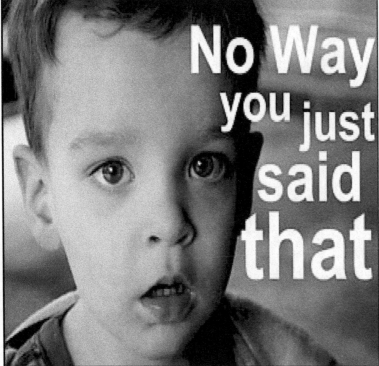

Sadly, when it comes to exercise, too many women are misguided or ill-informed. My "proof"? Just ask any of them WHY they attend exercise classes? Here are the top reasons you'll hear:

1 – "My Instructor Says I Can Burn 1000 Calories in Her Class!" The Truth: Being OVER-FAT is – and always will be – a "dietary issue". The amount of calories burned during exercise is grossly over-reported by the fitness industry. Is exercise important? Duh, of course it is. However, do it to be healthier and fitter, NOT to lose weight. Calories Calories Calories...

2 – "I'm Trying to Lose My Belly and Firm-up My Flabby Arms".
The Truth: Unless you understand the CAUSE AND EFFECT of EXERCISE, you may be NEEDLESSLY spinning your wheels engaged in an exercise program that will NEVER do what you want it to do. For years, I have seen (mostly) women jumping around - three-times per week - in a dance-type exercise class, and believing it is going to trim their waist, sculpt their flabby arms, and re-shape their fat asses. It will NOT! Often, one year later, I see those same people, still attending their favorite Exercise Instructor's class, and STILL FAT. Calories Calories Calories...

3 – "I LOST 30-Pounds Going to ZUMBA Classes... Hey, It WORKS For ME!"
The Truth: When people say, "Yeah, but it worked for me - it changed my body". No, your DIET changed your body. Your "classes" were simply fun. Rarely do I see FAT bodies - who regularly engage in Exercise Classes - change. Too many people (women mostly) believe that if they engage in an exercise class 3-4 times per, they are then doing their part to drop pounds. They are not. Exercise will NEVER cancel-out stuffing your face. Calories Calories calories....

Why Most Exercise Classes Are Filled with FAT People

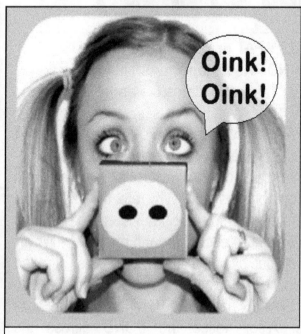

Oink! Oink!

4 – "I Joined a Gym Yesterday and Signed-up for "Butt-Buster" Classes".
The Truth: Again, lack of exercise knowledge is what allows gyms to sell their over-weight new members the "wrong" exercise prescription. That's "if" your goal is weight-loss, or a firmer more sculpted body, which is - according to the women, I speak with - the #1 goal of most women. You joined a new gym, that's great...exercise is good. You'll see your body change MOST quickly by engaging in strength-training, and at the same time, revamping your EATING habits. POW! **BOTTOM-LINE:** Whenever I present to groups, I always get a "huh?" response when I explain that exercise comes in many varieties. The one "you" choose to engage in on a regular basis can only DO what it is capable of doing, and it can NEVER do what it is NOT capable of doing." In other words, Zumba, Les Mills Videos, Cardio-Pump Classes, Boot Camps, etc., may in fact be "fun", and yes, that does have some value, but because these-type exercise programs can NOT be progressively more intense by-nature, and because it is impossible to measure the extent of the amount of (if any) progressive over-loading of the musculature, these become poor exercise choices if "results" is the goal. If Zumba or Brazilian Butt-Lift gets you motivated to exercise, so be it. Doing "something" will ALWAYS be better than doing NOTHING. Besides, it may be the gateway to other exercise-programs which are more productive, such as high-intensity strength training, which is "still" the most scientifically supported way to "CHANGE the WAY YOUR BODY LOOKS"; Second ONLY to REDUCING YOUR DAILY CALORIES. Note: My Exercise Instructors often think I am "scaring away business". I usually say, "No, I am NOT biased against anything, except "Lies and Myths". I explain the facts and where the evidence points. Your Customers or Clients can decide for themselves.

Why BELLY-FAT Seems So Stubborn (Think "Puddles & Ponds")

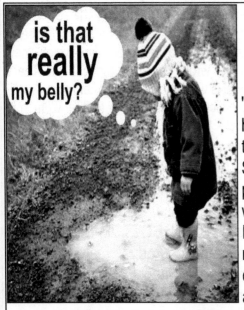

**BELLY-FAT or "LAST FEW POUNDS"
Are NOT As Stubborn As They Seem.
Think "Puddles & Ponds"**

"BELLY-FAT" always reminds me of a conversation I had years ago. Me and a group of friends were sitting on an outdoor deck after a Summer Rain Storm. Someone asked, "Why are those last few pounds of belly fat, so stubborn. I seem to be losing weight everywhere except around my waist - Why?" I said, look out over the deck, it has just stopped raining. Notice, the ground is now WET, and as you can see, WATER has pooled to form PUDDLES of all sizes. Also, notice the POND across the street...it has swelled to accommodate the newly deposited rain-WATER. Eventually, the SUN will appear and ALL the WATER will begin to evaporate. Our BODY-FAT is a lot like the rain water; hear me out. RAIN-WATER and BODY-FAT are similar because after a soaking rain storm, and as the sun appears, all the rain water will immediately begin to evaporate at the SAME rate...much like our own body-fat stores. However, to the naked-eye, it doesn't seem that way because although the ground dries very quickly, it may take until mid-day for the SMALLER PUDDLES to dry-up and be gone... The LARGER PUDDLES are shrinking too, yet it may actually take a full day or two for them to be dried-up and gone. Lastly, the POND across the street won't change much at all after only one day of sunshine"...but, I assure you, it's shrinking too. HERE'S THE GOOD PART: Our own "Body-fat" is a lot like the WET streets, PUDDLES, and POND. Much like the thin layer of water that covers the landscape, we all have a thin layer of fat accumulated underneath our skin over most of our bodies. It's called "Subcutaneous -Fat" (which simply means "under the skin"). We also store body-fat in larger quantities all around the body - kind of like PUDDLES. Doctors call this "Depot Fat". For women,

Why BELLY-FAT Seems So Stubborn (Think "Puddles & Ponds")

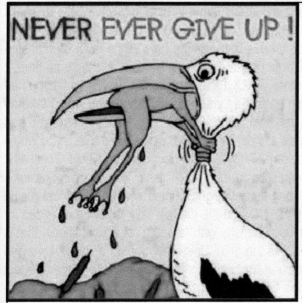

NEVER EVER GIVE UP !

FAT tends to gather in the biggest amounts on their hips, butt, and thighs. For men, it tends to gather on around their middle and lower back. These areas are our body's "Pond". The classic "Pond" on men of course, is what they jokingly refer to as their "beer belly". For women, their Pond is usually their butt or thighs. As we lose fat from exercise or reduced-calorie eating, the fat-loss in our body is like the evaporating water in the pond. Unfortunately, although the water is evaporating, it's not until the shoreline recedes, that we notice a water-level drop. Make sense? THE FRUSTRATING PART: Male Bodybuilders can relate to this concept from their own experiences with contest-dieting. Their Abs are the last area of their body to experience total leanness. This is because they begin their fat-loss diets with the most amount of fat (usually) around their middle. Female Bodybuilders would agree that it's usually their butt and upper-thighs that are the last to experience razor-sharp leanness. Therefore, if you are exercising and eating to lose fat, but seeing results only in some areas of your body and not others - DO NOT GET DISCOURAGED. Your belly-fat (or butt-fat) is NOT being stubborn at all. It's losing fat as fast as the rest of your body. It just seems like a slow poke because it's a "Pond", not a "wet street", or "puddle". Our bodies burn fat like the sun evaporates water on the town, a little at a time, but, ALL at the same time. Make sense? IMPORTANT NOTE: Performing extra abs exercises WILL NOT help. Remember, you can NOT spot reduce body-fat around your waist by exercising that area - that myth died long ago." Share this explanation with your own friends, 'cause most of them don't have a clue, and this explanation will help them keep their sanity during their own efforts to rid themselves of "those last few pounds".

"High- Intensity" Weight-Training Makes The Most Sense

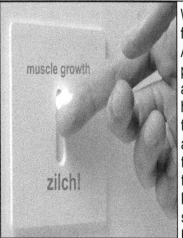
muscle growth

zilch!

Whenever I see muscle-heads in the gym doing countless sets or training for up to two-hours, and ask them "Why" they train this way, the answer I ALWAYS hear usually has something to do with training "hard." What people do NOT understand is that training hard (High level of intensity) and training long (1-2 hour workout), cannot be done at the same time; it has to be one or the other. PROOF? Think of it this way: If I said you had to run a 100-yard dash as fast as you possibly could, you would take-off at full-speed as soon as I said, "Go!" On the other hand, if I said you had to run 5-miles as fast as you possibly could, when I said "Go!", you would take-off at a much slower pace. Why? It is because you would "intuitively" know that in order to finish, you must pace itself. You can run fast for a short time, but not a long time. Weight training sessions that last for an hour or longer, simply will NOT be the intense "all-out" efforts needed for optimum training results. And by the way, do not confuse intensity with "amount" of weight lifted - that is another discussion. RESULTS? Whenever "RESULTS" is the goal, "intensity" should always be viewed as more important than "exercising longer". Again, that's if "getting as strong as possible in the shortest time possible" is truly your goal For most, it is. Muscles GROW or become stronger in response to training intensity, and only IF that intensity challenges your muscle's current capacity to perform work. In other words, it has to be demanding enough to feel as if it is the HARDEST you've ever worked. It is ONLY then, that an "Adaptive Response" within the muscle, takes place. Simply put, the body, through a number of metabolic processes, replenishes and repairs itself, and becomes stronger. Experts agree that this process normally takes between 48-96-hours. IMPORTANT NOTE: The reason for these seemingly wide "recovery" time-parameters is because of variable such as quality of rest, manual-labor jobs, genetics, etc. This is why scientist are unable to pin-point an exact number of hours for full-recovery. Perhaps the MOST compelling argument in-favor of the "One-Set" training protocol, is the research evidence that says that the adaptive response to "grow" actually happens within a muscle in a precise moment. Your intensity-of-effort either "trips" the adaptive response "switch" (like a light switch), or it does not. In addition, once it trips, you cannot trip it repeatedly in the same exercise session. In other words, ALL duplicated exercises performed (multiple sets) are nothing more than meaningless manual labor, i.e. a waste of your time. Furthermore, the extra sets will actually cause the muscles to require more recuperation time - you know it as over-training - sound familiar? Not only does credible exercise-science support the one-set training protocol, but most of today's informed weight-training professionals no longer recommend multiple-set training protocols to their clients. The biggest mistake I see women who weight train make, is NOT training intensely enough - as if it was exclusively a "man's thing", to train hard. The best "tip" a woman in the gym will EVER get, is to engage in high-intensity strength-training.

Another Reason to Choose High-Intensity Training

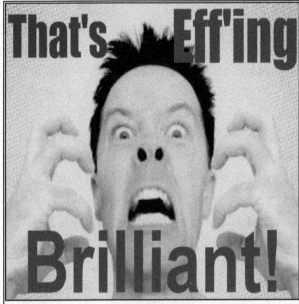

By now, most informed fitness professionals know that High Intensity Training is the most scientifically-supported training method for its ability to produce "results". Therefore, there's no sense beating that subject to death. But, perhaps the best reason to engage in High Intensity Training has nothing to do with how quickly it produces results. The greatest benefits of high intensity training may be what it DOES NOT Do. High Intensity Training is the most TIME-EFFICIENT. Therefore, it DOES NOT take up much of your time. Why spend 1-2 hours in the gym, when you can get the same or better results approximately 30-minutes or LESS? No Brainer. High Intensity Training DOES NOT pound the hell out of your joints, therefore it is the SAFEST type of training. Although strenuous, because it is performed in a slow-controlled manner, there is virtually no risk of muscle, tendon, ligament, or joint injury, due to ballistic, joint-jarring movements. Again, a No Brainer. High Intensity Training DOES NOT make you pay later for being an Idiot. It is the forgiving type of training. Knuckle-heads, who perform countless sets - five, six, or even seven days per-week, should ask anybody who has spent their lives performing manual labor, just what it does to their bodies later in life. It beats the hell out of their joints – they simply wear out. Arthritic-type issues later in life are almost a certainty. This is exactly where the average high-volume weight training enthusiast is headed. Once again, a No Brainer. Your genetics "will" largely determine your body's response to training, and therefore, your end results. But, whatever results you are destined to achieve, wouldn't it make the "most" sense to achieve them in the "shortest" time possible, and with the "least chance" of injury, and with the "smallest amount" of wear n' tear on your body?" High Intensity Training is and always will be, a No Brainer.

The REAL Reason Why Women Must Lift Weights

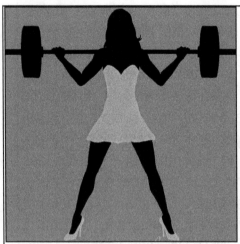

Ladies, Ask Yourself This: Does your naked body at-40 look anything like it did, at 20...even though you may even still "weigh about the same?" For most, the answer is "No". Want to know why? The answer would surprise MOST ladies; It's their LOSS of MUSCLE MASS! Women, it's time to say "Yes" to weight-training. I know what you're thinking: **"I don't want big muscles!" (duh) - "I don't want to look like a bodybuilder!" (double duh) - "I actually want smaller muscles!" (Oh brother).** For the last time, it's time to put this myth to rest. Women should NOT shy away from weight-training (a.k.a. resistance training or strength training). It is essential to remaining youthful, and having the lean, toned, and shapely body - you want so badly. Myth Busted: "Lifting-weights makes women "bulky". Nonsense! A women's unfavorable genetic factors, such as lack of testosterone, levels of estrogen, cross section width of muscle bellies, etc., simply precludes 99.9% of woman from getting "big muscles" - blah, blah, blah - but it's true! **The Facts:** As women age (men too), their muscle mass decreases – it is a natural process of aging. Losing as little as one-half pound of muscle can result in additional fat deposits on your butt and thighs. Why? Because muscle is active tissue, which makes high calorie demands - even when you're lying in bed at night. Less muscle means a slower resting-metabolism. As early as your middle 20's, the average woman experiences a slight decline in her metabolic rate each year, which exactly parallels her loss of muscle mass. The relationship is obvious: as muscle-mass decreases, metabolism slows. As a woman ages – even if she continues to eat the same number of calories per day – she gets fatter and fatter. Plain n' simply, the loss of muscle equals a decline in metabolic rate. And, it gets worse year after year. **The Truth Hurts:** The passage of time (alone) puts ALL women on the road to eventually having an over-fat and out-of-shape body. Yes, an older is probably going to be a FATTER you (wait n' see). Weight training is the #1 way to slow or stop this natural aging process. It's not a matter of building bigger muscles, you should be exercising simply to KEEP the Muscles you have now. By the way, it is NEVER to late to start.

Free-Weights Or Machines?

The age-old debate, which is better: *free weights or machines?* The fact of the matter is, they both have their own unique advantages. However, one myth that needs to be put to rest is that free-weights are best for putting-on "size", while machines are more for "toning". This is simply untrue. Muscles don't know the difference between 50-lbs. of iron, or 50-lbs. of feathers. Muscles are actually quite dumb - they simply respond to the imposed physical-demand we place on them. One of the advantages of today's exercise-machines and cable-contraptions do have over free-weights, is allowing resistance to be applied to a working-muscle through its entire range-of-motion. The best example being the "Pec-dec" (Chest Fly machine) vs. Chest-flies performed with two-dumbbells. In addition, machines have an advantage for being more time-efficient (pin-selection vs. unloading plates) and safety (the weight usually travels on a fixed-plane of movement and rarely requires the use of a "spotter"). My "Free-weight" friends would probably counter with the fact that it takes more "balance" to bench-press a barbell. The truth is they are correct. In the case of bench-pressing, the shoulder muscles must contract as stabilizers to keep the arms from flailing-about as the primary-muscles – the chest, front-delts, and triceps – perform the movement. Another example is the barbell squat, which takes many more muscle groups to balance and stabilize the body as opposed to a leg-press machine. All factors considered, I personally give the advantage to machines over free-weights. With advanced ergonomic planes of movement and variable resistance able to be applied to the entire range of motion, emphasizing maximum load in the strongest contracted position, today's machines are more advantageous in so many ways. However, as I stated in the beginning, BOTH free-weights and exercise-machines can produce a safe and effective workout session when used properly. That said, outstanding physiques can certainly be built with free weights alone. Where this argument gets a bit tricky, is when it is argued that free-weights, because of the "balance" factor, is better when training for -say - "sports". This is not true, yet is widely believed. The skill of one is NOT necessarily transferable to sports movements. This is the faulty premise of the that some "Functional Training" programs are predicated on. Many athlete are engaging in workout regimens that have NOTHING to do improving their golf-swing or agility on the basketball court. Yet, I see athletes performing idiotic and nonsensical exercises all the time (That's another discussion). The bottom line is that in many ways, it comes down to personal preference, or working with what's available.

You Should Only Be Doing "Smart" Cardio

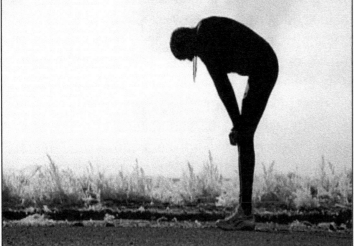

..Shoulda drove

The word "Cardio" means different thing to different people. For some, it's a leisurely walk, perhaps with a friend, to "get some exercise". For others, it's a blistering Treadmill or Elliptical Machine workout that has you out of breath in no time flat. Yet for others it's somewhere in the middle. So who's right? Allow me to explain. For anyone who has been bed-ridden for months, a walk down the driveway to their mailbox may indeed feel like a cardio-workout.

Here's my point: Let's not get caught-up in the "aerobic" vs. "anaerobic" discussion. Anybody attempting to change the way their body looks is going to have their own "starting-point", regarding how fit they are in this precise moment. This becomes their own personal "Square-One". With this in-mind, you must now chose an activity to "start" with. The key is, it has to be something that you can do for 20-30 minutes, that will challenge your current cardio-vascular fitness level. In-other-words, it has to be at least mildly uncomfortable to complete, yet, attainable. For example: Let's say, you are extremely sedentary, so for you, "walking" would be a good place to start. Go out for a 20-minute or-so walk. Challenge yourself a bit...but at this point, since you're not used to exercise of any kind - don't push it too much. Okay, that's it! You will now do this on 3 non-consecutive days per-week (e.g. Mon-Wed-Fri). This is the important part; every time you go for your walk, constantly challenge yourself to cover more ground in the same 20-30 minutes. In-other-words, instead of increasing the minutes you spend walking, spend those same number of minutes attempting to travel further. You may want to eventually alternate your pace between power-walking

You Should Only Be Doing "Smart" Cardio

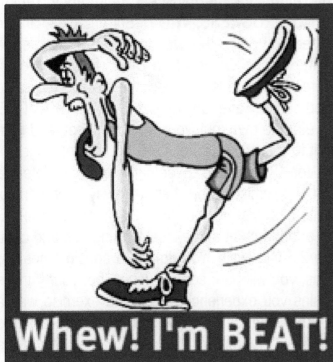

Whew! I'm BEAT!

and recovery-walking...anything to cover more distance. Build up to run-walk intervals, then from there, perhaps "all" running. There is a very important reason why you should do it this way. Increasing your fitness-level, becoming stronger, or burning more fat, is always going to involve increasing your level of "intensity" of effort. This will ALWAYS allow us to get the most results out of exercise in the shortest amount of time. Otherwise, if we kept trying to exercise longer...where does it end? Does 30-minutes soon turn into an hour?...then eventually 2 or 3 hours? This is neither time-efficient - who the hell has all day to exercise - nor the best way to get stronger or fitter. Not to mention it will probably save you a ton of needless wear n' tear on your joints. Your knees will thank you later in life. You should NEVER aspire to run or jog for an excessive amount of miles. The only exception is if you are (or want to be) an athlete that competes at running. Again, unless you are a competitive "Long-distance Runner", this training protocol makes little sense. This form of exercise has been long-abandoned by most top athletes of the world. It robs the body of lean tissue (emaciated-runner syndrome), has long-term repetitive-use-injury ramification (pounds the hell out of knee and ankle joints), modern athletes have replaced over-distance-running with more efficient "interval-type" training (Heck, even marathon runner do not log the excessive training miles that were customary in the 70's and 80's). These days, High School Football players doing countless "laps" around the field for conditioning purposes is the sign of an uneducated Coach.

The "Ground Hog Day" Exercise Rut

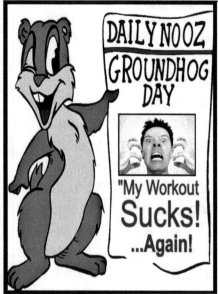

DAILY NOOZ
GROUNDHOG DAY

"My Workout Sucks! ...Again!"

"I'm Following My Workout Sheet Religiously, Yet I'm Making NO PROGRESS, Why?" Sorry Ladies - In the gym - I see you doing this way too often. It makes me think of the movie "Ground Hog Day?" In other words, your exercise session is similar to the movie - the same exact workout, day after day after day... FOR EXAMPLE: You arrive at the gym, pull your workout sheet, and then perform it to a tee; one set of THIS for 12 reps...one set of THAT for 12 reps, etc. Eventually, you complete the entire list of exercises. You then file-away your workout sheet until next visit to the gym. (Another) EXAMPLE: You and a friend meet at the local walking trial and complete the 2.5-mile walk. You do this a couple times per week. Yes, you will burn some calories, but your "fitness level" will not improve past the initial gains you experienced when the exercise was a "new" activity. Here's WHY Your PROGRESS Has STOPPED: You are simply failing to follow the most fundamental law of exercise, "Progressive Workload". Whether you are training with weights, walking, or jogging for exercise. Your body's fitness level will only improve, IF you place a demand on it that challenges its' current capacity to perform work. For example, the first time you ever performed a set of -say - "leg extensions", using 30 lbs., it was difficult to complete, therefore, on your rest-day, your body had an adaptive response to this workload - it got stronger... So, the next time you performed the same exercise, if you performed the same exercise, using the same amount of weight, and for the same number of repetitions, it DID NOT challenge your body's capacity for work. You now are performing work (exercise) that was well within your body's capabilities - therefore, NO adaptive response needed - NO progress. What About CARDIO? Same Thing Applies: If you walk 2.5 miles in 35 minutes, day-in and day-out, your body will adapt to this and eventually it will not improve your cardiovascular fitness level. YOU MUST challenge your body's current work-capacity, by (say) performing the same walk in a faster time, or by increasing the distance walked - one or the other. The BIG LESSON LEARNED: You MUST constantly challenge your body's current capacity to perform work. This is the KEY TO IMPROVEMENT in ALL your EXERCISE EFFORTS.

FOR MEN ONLY!
How HUGE Can You Really Get?

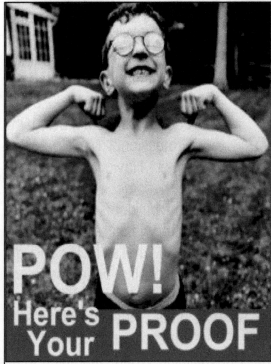

POW!
Here's Your PROOF

Skinny Gym-Dude: "Hey Man, What's The Best Workout For Getting HUGE?"

Huge Gym-Dude: "Blah, Blah, Blah, Blah, Blah..." For starter, it is WRONG to assume that someone's "exercise" knowledge or credibility is predicated on "how they look". If it were that simple, why don't we just ask the biggest bodybuilder in the world, "How they got so big", and then follow it, verbatim. See what I mean? It's like the average-looking woman asking the beautiful girl they see at the mall, "Tell me how to become beautiful, so I can be too?" Sorry, it doesn't work that way. WHY you should not necessarily believe your local gym's muscle-head's training advice: Most "future" bodybuilding greats had to - like you - begin as a skinny novice. The difference is, "they" suddenly realize that they have a great genetic-predisposition for muscle-growth. How? They start growing like crazy! For them, it's easy to get great muscle-building results from even the most idiotic training routines. Moreover, they ACTUALLY BELIEVE that it's the supplements they're taking, or idiotic (outdated) training methods that are responsible for their success, when in fact NOTHING could be further from the truth. The truth is, most guys beating the hell out of their bodies in the gym just don't understand that developing "freaky" muscle-size and strength is predicated on 3-factors. Here they are in the order of importance:

1 - GENETICS. The dudes in the Muscle Magazines (Mr. Olympia Competitors) have one huge advantage: They are blessed with genetics that belong to only One-Thousandth of 1% of the men in the United States. Do the math, chances are it's not you - sorry, sometimes the truth is hard to swallow...better you learn it now.

Grrrrr....

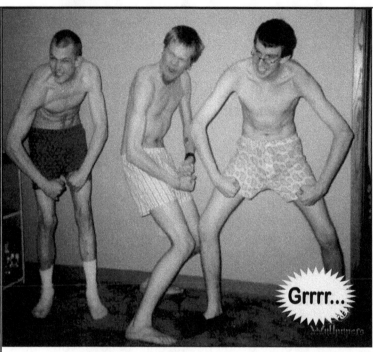

Grrrr...

2 - STEROIDS. No matter what ANYBODY tells you, the combination of Genetics and Anabolic Drugs is the ONLY way to produce the bodies we see gracing the Professional Muscle Magazines. Having the genetics to become a Mr. Olympia bodybuilder is as rare as the lottery-jackpot odds...and even that's NOT enough. You'd also better be ready to take steroids by the truckloads. Anybody that says genetics and training hard works too; I offer you this: Compare a "Natural" Bodybuilding World Champion to an IFBB Champion; Case closed. It's like Pee-wee Herman standing next to King Kong.

3 - WORKOUT REGIMEN. Trust me, when it comes to being on the cover of your favorite Muscle-Magazine, the way you "train" is a very distant 3rd to genetics and steroids - Just sayin'.'. That's why most guys who do "everything" correctly, still can't be Mr. America. Conversely, this is also why some people who do the dumbest things in the gym, still look great. Read the sections that explains "High-Intensity" for the best ways to develop strength. Evidence-based training principles will always be the most logical way to exercise. All you can hope to contribute your aspirations of having HUGE MUSCLES is to use evidence-based strength-training principles (Brief, high-intensity workouts). And then, let the chips will fall where-they-may. The lack of understand of human-genetics is so prevalent among gym idiots - we will continue to have this argument, over, and over, and over...

Your "Bodybuilding Heroes" Were WRONG!

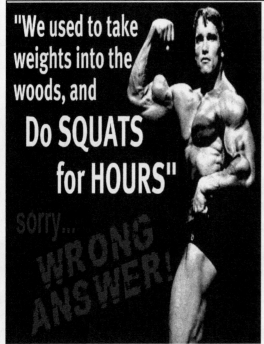

"We used to take weights into the woods, and **Do SQUATS for HOURS**" sorry... WRONG ANSWER!

Train Like "Johnny Big Arms" and you'll soon have arms as big as Johnny's, right? Wrong. I have had this argument with my gym buddies hundreds of times over the years. They just can't wrap their (muscle) heads around the notion that many of their bodybuilding heroes were (are) able to develop an awesome body IN-SPITE of their workout routine, and not BECAUSE of their workout routine. No offense to the great Arnold Schwarzenegger, but the truth is, great genetics can (and does) cover-up a lot of stupid training-habits. Guys Always Say, *"But, I'll Do ANYTHING To Get H-U-G-E!"* This is the exact reason it is SO easy to fall for Supplement Ads. When most guys - and this applies to 99.99% of all aspiring muscle-heads - realize that they are just NOT getting as HUGE as they'd like, their first reaction is to wonder *"What supplement am I missing?"*, Or, *"Am I training long enough?"* Of course this a "perfect storm" of faulty-thinking because there is a long line of pretty-faced Fitness Models and Mega-Muscled Goons waiting to SELL you some good-for-nothing product, which promises; *"You Can Look Like Me!"* Sorry, you can't, and probably won't. Believe it or not, most of today's informed weight-training professionals actually shake their heads and laugh at Arnold Schwarzenegger's training habits. This of course goes for many of the muscle magazine cover gods, who really owe their bodybuilding success to lottery-winning genetics, and an truck-load of steroids. You may feel like asking, *"Are You Trying to Shatter My Muscle-Building Dreams?"* Nope. Far from it. I'm simply advocating for evidence-based high-intensity strength training, which just happens to be MOST productive anyway. My question to you is, Why not get as big and strong as you can, as quickly as you can? Instead, many are NOT realizing the heights of their muscle-building potential because they keep switching up from one stupid and dumb way of training to another. As for the supplements? Hey look, I'm simply trying to stop you from wasting a ton of money. I get it; Johnny Big Arms is a LOT more convincing than I am. Hey, you can decide for yourself.

Want BIGGER Muscles? STOP Training (Say Wut!)

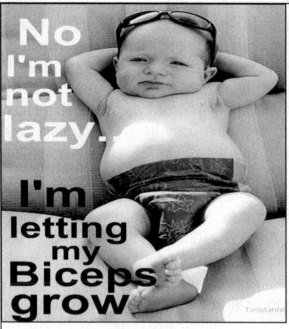

No I'm not lazy.. I'm letting my Biceps grow

Most workout enthusiast should realize that as hard as they train, ANY WORKOUT is only as good as your ability to recover from it. Sometimes a "DAY-OFF" is the BEST thing you can do, to make your muscles BIGGER and STRONGER. When a muscle is put through a workout, and the proper amount of training-stimulus occurs, it then takes 48-96 hours to fully-recover and allow an adaptive-response to occur (I.e. get stronger). If you do not allow this process-chain to fully occur, you will find yourself making no-measurable progress from your workouts, or worse, sliding backwards or losing strength. Making a muscle grow as quickly as possible has as much to do with "rest", as it does with intense training. Many of my bodybuilding buddies perform split-routines. They're in the gym 6-7 days-per-week training different muscles on different days. What's hard to get through their thick heads is that recovery-ability is not only "muscle-specific", but also "systemic". When you blast through a chest or leg workout, not only are those targeted muscles greatly taxed and in-need of rest, but so is your central-nervous system. When a person trains intensely for 6 out-of-the 7 days in a week, even though they may argue "yeah, but I'm training different muscles", they are often NOT allowing the trained-muscle to recover, because the recovery-ability needed is being used-up by constant daily expenditure on all your other muscles too. Again, this is so common with "split-routines" that are so popular with ill-informed aspiring bodybuilders. **It's hard to replace "More is Better" thinking, with "Less is Best"...but it is. Knowing my muscle-head friends as well as I do, somehow I know they're NOT listening ...Grrrrrr**

WHY Do Men Cheat? (At Exercise)

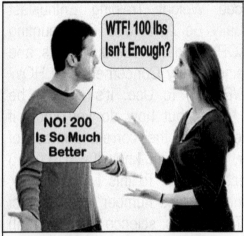

The law of physics state that, "an object in motion tends to stay in motion." Well, ego-driven gym-dudes figured this out a long time ago. In the gym, guys look so silly when they jerk, swing, or throw weights around. Do they even realize that "acceleration and momentum" is what's lifting most of the weight? Suddenly they are able to lift (say) 200 lbs. instead of 100 lbs. What they don't realize is that instead of looking like Hercules - to the "informed" observer - they look more like an idiot. Here are two major reasons WHY you should NOT fall for the temptation to throw and swing the weights you are lifting:

1 – LESS TRAINING RESULTS: The true Irony is that momentum actually takes away from the training effect of the exercise. The longer the time that momentum is actually lifting the weight - instead of your muscles - the lesser the training-effect of the exercise. Therefore, you are not increasing your strength-level in the fastest time possible. Again, what irony.

2 – JOINT DAMAGE: Momentum causes much-greater stress on the joints, bones, tendons, and ligaments involved. Not only is there an immediate injury risk, but if this type of stress is placed on body-parts regularly, you may escape injury in the short-term, but long-term, don't be surprised if your "joints" hate you for it. If you don't believe that repetitive high-impact jarring of the joints is going to catch-up with you. Just ask any former NFL Football Player who is now in their 50's or 60's.

3 - Simple: You'll Look Like an IDIOT!

The Bottom Line: "Poor Exercise Form" is the most common mistake taking place in most gyms. Perform each repetition in a slow and controlled manner. This is the most effective way to increase muscle-strength and muscle-size. Yes, you probably have to use less weight than usual. Don't worry, you will soon be properly lifting the same amount of weight that you used to throw around. Look on the bright side; now the people in the gym that "do" know what the hell they're doing, will no-longer look at you and say, **"LOOK AT THAT IDIOT!"**

How MUCH Weight? How MANY Reps?

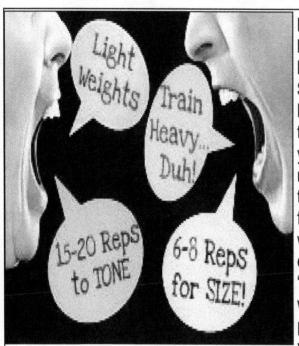

Experienced Weight Training Enthusiast May Actually Be Able to STOP Counting Reps, STOP Filling out Workout Charts, and STOP Being Overly Concerned With HOW MUCH WEIGHT To Use. It's easy to be thinking, "Okay, but how do you know if you're performing the correct number of reps?" Or, "How do you know if you're using the correct weight?" To this I would reply, first define "correct number", or "correct weight? The truth is, science and the (real) experts have NEVER really figured-out the "exact number" of reps, or the "exact weight" we should all be using…and they probably never will. There are just too many variables existing from person to person. Instead, the experts agree on "parameters". In other words, they agree that it's somewhere between "here" and "there"…and there's a lot of latitude, which makes the so-called targeted number (of reps and weight) pretty easy to hit. The real purpose of repetitions is to allow a targeted muscle to perform physical work continuously for an optimal amount of time to stimulate an adaptive response (get bigger and stronger). That amount of time is between 35-seconds and 90-seconds, depending "which" expert you ask. In terms of "reps", these time parameters equal somewhere between 8-20 strict repetitions being the targeted number. Again, that's a wide and therefore pretty easy target to hit. The thing ALL qualified experts DO agree on is that the 2 MOST IMPORTANT exercise criteria to increase strength or stimulating muscle growth are: **1 - You MUST exercise at a high enough level of intensity, which means you MUST reach a point of maximal effort during such exercise. By the way, It's a mistake to confuse "heavy weight" with intensity. 2 - You MUST exercise in a manner which is progressively more difficult to perform and therefore challenges your current maximum capacity to perform work (i.e. Progressive Overload).** So, you may be thinking:

How MUCH Weight? How MANY Reps?

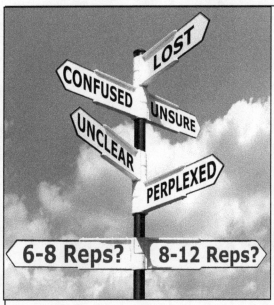

"What does this have to do with never having to count reps, get overly concerned about choosing the correct weight; or not having to write down the weight and/or reps?" That's easy. Say, you are on vacation and decided to hit the weight-room at your resort. Again we're talking about a person who's been working out with weights for a reasonable amount of time. You walk over to (say) the Lat-Pull-down machine. Not knowing the machine, most experienced lifters would just arbitrarily select a weight, and then perform a "test rep" or two. Based on your experience and knowing your own body, you would probably be able to immediately (and intuitively) assess if the weight was a bit too light, a bit too heavy, or just right...Now, after making any necessary weight adjustment, let's say you then strictly performed as many repetitions as physically possible. Because you performed the exercise to a point of momentary muscular familiar, it's then a certainty that you reached an appropriate level of "intensity", and performed the work to the limit of your own physical abilities. Therefore the exercise would be "both", intense enough and progressive enough to produce an adaptive response within the working muscle. As long as the weight wasn't ridiculously too light or too heavy, does it really matter how much weight you used, or how many reps you performed? Not really. Again, it's because the target number of both is wide, therefore pretty easy to hit. The next time you go to the gym, instead of using a machine you are familiar with - try a new one. Make an educated guess at the starting weight, try a test rep or two to confirm, make the adjustment (or not), and then perform - in strict form - as many reps as physically possible. If you do this, there's a 99% chance that you will have met ALL the criteria to make that muscle grow and become stronger. Using this training protocol, you will continue to get stronger, and experience a variety in training that will help you avoid staleness or training plateaus. Give it a try!

Chapter 4

Things Even "Smart People" STILL Get Wrong

Eating LESS vs. Exercising MORE Which is Best?

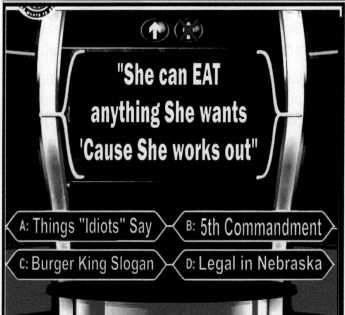

"She can EAT anything She wants 'Cause She works out"

A: Things "Idiots" Say
B: 5th Commandment
C: Burger King Slogan
D: Legal in Nebraska

Whenever I hear somebody say, "SHE CAN EAT ANYTHING SHE WANTS, 'CAUSE SHE WORKS-OUT", I always think to myself, "Wrong answer!" Exercising is NOT capable of canceling-out regularly Stuffing Your Face - no matter HOW MUCH you exercise. Here's Why: The amount of calories burned in even the most strenuous exercise session is not nearly as much as most people think. A few hundred calories (at most) is all that you'll burn. Even if Exercise Instructors want to throw in the "Exercise After-Burn" argument, they will STILL lose this argument. You can easily wipe-out the calories-burned in an hour of exercise with a low-fat yogurt or a few handfuls of nuts - and these are "good foods". Here's the proof: Let's say you had the physical ability to run for 24-hours straight without stopping. Anybody would agree that this would certainly boost your body's calorie-burning, right? Okay, follow along; On this 24-hour run, let's say you fueled your body by eating a constant supply of apples. It takes about 3-minutes to eat a medium sized apple. Therefore, for 24-hours, you are continuously running while eating an apple at the rate of about one every 3 minutes. QUESTION: "Does the constant supply of apples you'd be eating provide enough calories/energy to fuel your body to run non-stop for 24-hours?" ANSWER: Not only is the answer "Yes", the truth is, you would actually GAIN 6 lbs. of BODY FAT (Do the math). My point is that I would hate to see anyone begin an exercise-routine, only to find themselves spinning their wheels - making no progress, all because they haven't given "food-intake" its proper priority. WEIGHT-LOSS will ALWAYS be about REDUCING YOUR CALORIE IN-TAKE. The BEST WEIGHT-LOSS RESULTS are accomplished by reducing your calorie-intake. And then, for reasons having more to do with physical appearance and good health, by all means, EXERCISE!

Do "Genetics" Really Matter?

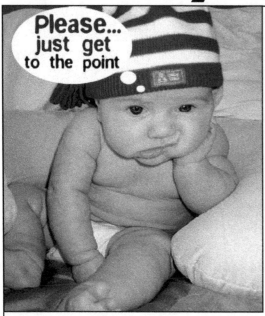

Please... just get to the point

Science can be a bit boring, so let's address the basics - once and for all.

Genetics: The inherited physical characteristics passed onto you from your parents and their gene-pool. You can actually inherit traits from any of your ancestors. For some, it's like winning the lottery (good genes). For others, it's like being cursed (not so good genes). Like it or not, you can be "fated" to be fat. Without delving into too much complicated science, it may help to have at least a basic understanding of what Scientist refer to as the 3-Basic "Somatotypes": Endomorph, Ectomorph, and Mesomorph. In-other-word, the 3-types of "builds" you can be born with. Can you identify your own body-type?

The "Endomorph": Characterized by round and curvy features and naturally possessing a larger amount of body-fat than other body-types. The fat is predominately distributed on the lower body; the belly, hips, butt, and thighs. The Endomorph is the body-type most likely to experience obesity. The good news? It's not as bad as it seems. You can have an endomorphic body and still look great. Actresses, Marilyn Monroe, Jennifer Lopez (J-Lo), and singer, Beyoncé', are past and present examples of endomorphic-type bodies that achieved sex-symbol status in Hollywood. Although the Endomorph is the most likely body-type to be sporting a few extra pounds, your "lifestyle" can be the great equalizer.

The "Ectomorph": Best described by one word -"Slim". Long slender limbs and difficulty gaining weight (it's okay to be a little jealous), describes the Ectomorph, perfectly. The most obvious example being of course - Fashion and

Do "Genetics" Really Matter?

Runway Models. Men and women with this body-type, naturally having lower levels of lean muscle-mass - which give the body it's shapeliness - may want to make "resistance-training" part of their lifestyle.

The "Mesomorph": Two word often describe this body-type - "Muscular" and "Athletic". Wide at the shoulders and narrow at the hips. If you're a Mesomorph, you're probably the envy of all the gym-rats. You are naturally well-muscled, and possess a natural athletic build. In many ways, the Mesomorph is like genetic lottery winner! Mesomorphs have very little to complain about. Although science identifies and describes these specific body-types, in reality, most people can be - and actually are - a combination of more than one body-type. For example, you may possess a mesomorph upper-body and an ectomorph lower body. This is the dilemma of many Male Bodybuilders. They sport a thickly muscled upper-body, yet have a more stick-figure lower-body. Female Bodybuilders often face a different body-type dilemma because it's common among females to actually possess an ectomorph upper-body, and an endomorphic lower-body. This is characterized by disproportionately-large hips, butt, and thighs, while possessing an upper-body displays little body-fat. It creates a very frustrating "weight-training" dilemma for each.

Note: Genetic factors are discussed in this book because they "do" matter . We ALL must play the (genetic) hand we're dealt. You can't reasonably expect to ever be mistaken for a petite Ballerina if you were born with a body-type more common to an NFL Linebacker...Sorry. However, although genetics cannot be totally cancelled-out as a factor in how your body looks in the mirror, the good-news is, the image that is staring back at you is more reflective of the "lifestyle" you lead. 25% of a person's body-weight is determined by Genetics - The other 75% is determined by their Lifestyle. When someone says "Genetics don't matter", they're either clueless, or, trying to sell you something.

"Will BUTT EXERCISE Make My FLAT BUTT, Round?"

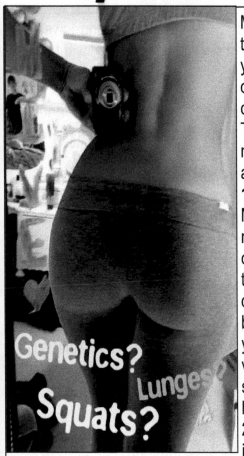

My personal favorite muscle-shape-myth is that certain "Butt Exercises" can make a Flat Butt, round. For years, bodybuilders believed that doing a certain type of Bicep-Curl would add a "peak" to their biceps? Of course, credible-science proved this to be false. The TRUTH is, when you look at your Naked-Butt in the mirror, there 2-FACTORS that determines how pleasant - or unpleasant - the reflecting image is.

1 - GENETICS: The actual SHAPE of your Glute Muscles is determined solely by your Genetics. Remember, your Butt is a "Muscle", just like your biceps, calves, quads, etc. It's SHAPE is inherent and unique to you specifically. If you train your Glutes – like you do other muscles – it will become stronger and grow, but its shape will not change. In other words, whether you naturally possess a round-type Butt or a flatter-version, you probably ALWAYS will - you'll just possess a stronger or more developed Butt. No matter how much we want this to NOT be true, it IS.

2 - BODY-FAT: on your Butt is the other major factor in determining its physical-appearance. More importantly, this you CAN change. Yes, if and when you reduce the globs of fat on your Butt, curves will suddenly begin to appear. Look at it this way; If you were to take a granite-statue of a perfectly sculpted human-body, and then, take handfuls of clay and begin to slap it one the statue, eventually the nooks n' crannies of the sculpted granite would be filled with clay, causing the statue to look more like the Michelin Man than a Greek God or Goddess. BODY-FAT has the same effect on your Butt's physical-appearance. It robs your Butt of some - or all - of its shape by filling in your muscle's nook n' crannies much like the clay added to the statue. **BOTTOM-LINE:** If you eat wisely and exercise intelligently, you won't be able to ever change the shape of your SHAPE of your Butt. However, by reducing body-fat levels the appearance of its shape WILL eventually change.

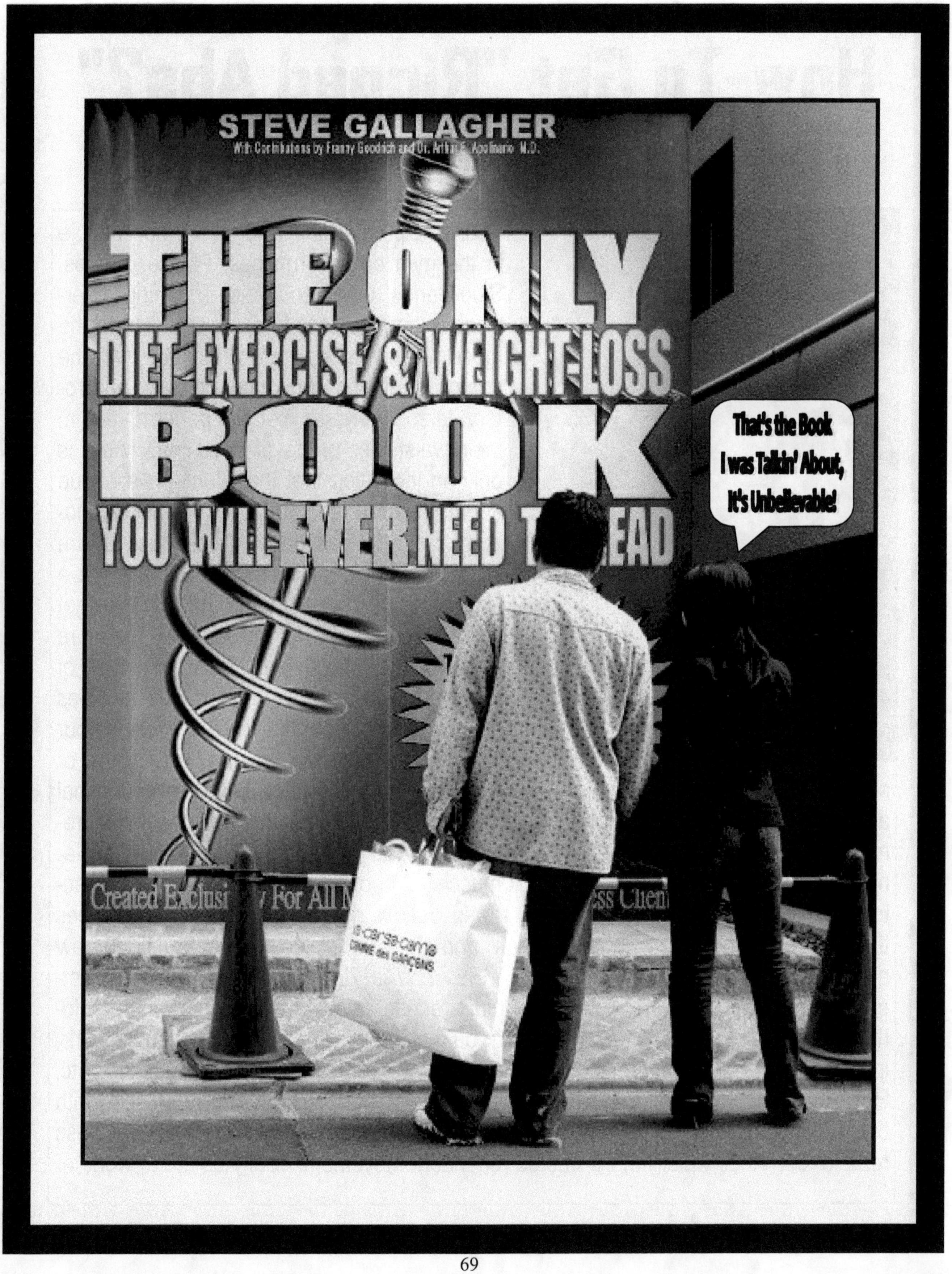
STEVE GALLAGHER
THE ONLY
DIET EXERCISE & WEIGHT-LOSS
BOOK
YOU WILL EVER NEED
That's the Book
I was Talkin' About,
It's Unbelievable!

How-To Get "Ripped Abs?" The Biggest LIE in Fitness

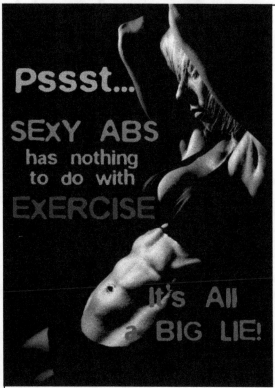

I can't help chuckling whenever I see people in the gym doing Crunches, Planks, Sit-ups, Side-Bends, or other "Waist Trimming" exercises. When it comes to exercise, Abs are the most misunderstood part of the body. All the crunches, sit-ups, trunk curls, planks, and rotary torso exercises people perform to trim their waist-line, or develop six-pack Abs, is only an indication that they don't have a clue about exercise and/or fat-loss. Nobody, nobody, nobody, has flabby Abs! Muscles are NEVER flabby. Flab is flabby! There is not a single exercise on this earth that will ever get rid of belly fat. The fat on your body is more about calorie-intake than about what type of exercises you do. Remember, Abs muscles are no different from any other muscle in your body. When exercised, muscles either grow or stay the same. You cannot "trim" a muscle. If anything, the muscles of the abdominal area will grow (slightly) when trained - meaning they actually increase the measurement of your waistline. Don't worry, without boring you with a lengthy physiology explanation, just know that the Abs and trunk muscles do not possess the physiological factors to experience much growth when strenuously worked - much like facial muscles that DO NOT grow when we chew, chew, and chew on a piece of steak until our jaw aches. YES, YOU CAN HAVE A LEAN & SEXY WAISTLINE! It's NOT that complicated...most people just don't "get-it." You must reduce calorie-intake or burn more calories by moving-more to melt away fat. So, you may be thinking, "should I even be working my Abs?" Sure! Strong Abs helps reduce low-back stress, improve posture, etc. However, remember, you should work your Abs as you would any other muscle, with brief, intense resistance exercise, period. Folks seem to think they need to do countless reps to "trim" their waistline; it's wasted redundant movement. Your Abs are at work for

...And, Why Exercise Does NOT "Melt" Body-Fat

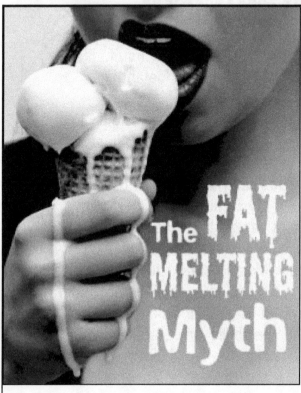

The FAT MELTING Myth

most of your waking day; walking, bending, twisting, and even sitting keeps them continuously contracting in-concert. Also, realize that whenever you are lifting anything heavy, forceful exhaling involves forceful isometric contractions of all abdominal muscles. In addition, anytime the body braces itself, as in over-head lifting, or pulling movements, the abdominal muscles - again - forcefully contract. Stop wasting your time performing hundreds of sit-ups or crunches - It DOESN'T WORK! While we're on the subject; Just because we feel a "burning" sensation in our muscles when we exercise, it is easy to make what seems to be a logical assumption, that "burning" must mean, "melting" – as in body fat melting away. Sorry, it doesn't work that way. Without going into a lengthy explanation about the physiological impossibility of "spot-reducing", which you can learn all about in some of my other posts, just trust me, all the abs-crunches and side-twists we all do to trim our mid-sections is virtually a waste of time. For all the bodybuilders out there laughing at the "clueless" – you're NO better. When it comes time for competition preparation, you ALL start doing tons of additional Abs-Crunches, Twists, and Side-Bends. Why? Again, it's mostly because it is so easy to be sucked-in to the false notion that burning muscles equals melting fat. Of course, it is no coincidence that the "Spot-Reducing" myth is one of the most profitable fitness "Lies," ever! I wonder how many people reading this are nodding their head in agreement, yet tomorrow in the gym will go right back to trying to slim or trim their own waist-line by bombarding it with "reps".

An EASY Way To Understand Your "Metabolism"

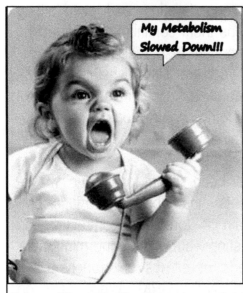

My Metabolism Slowed Down!!!

"It's NOT My Fault, I have a Slow Metabolism!"

"Really, I went on a Diet, and it SLOWED -DOWN My Metabolism!"

"No Really, As Soon as I Turned 40, My Metabolism STOPPED!"

Unfortunately, these remarks are usually made by people who do not understand what "Metabolism" actually is. The first thing we should understand about our metabolism is that it isn't just one tangible thing. It's actually the sum of all the metabolic processes and chemical-reactions in your body. For example: Digestion is a metabolism; cell-repair is a metabolism; burning calories in a working muscle is a metabolism; and so on. Every one of these "metabolisms" uses calories as energy to carry-out its unique task. Your "Resting-Metabolism" is simply the number of calories required to keep your body functioning when you're flopped on the sofa or snoozing. Your metabolism is actually burning calories continuously and without interruption, 24-hours per day; If it stopped - you'd be DEAD! DON'T GET CONFUSED, because the MOST IMPORTANT (and only) metabolism to concern yourself with is the metabolism that takes place in your MUSCLES. This is important in weight-loss for this reasons: Muscles, even at rest, consume the largest number of calories in our bodies. And better yet, these same muscles when "moving", consume calories at a multiplied rate, and it adds up quickly in your favor (fat-loss). Often, Supplement "Sellers" would like you to believe that certain foods - or diet supplements their selling - will "boost" your metabolism. This is bullshit. As previously noted, the digestion of ANY food "is" in-of-itself a me-

An EASY Way To Understand Your "Metabolism"

tabolism. When we eat food, it goes through a digestive process. It takes calories to perform this digestive process. Science refers to this as the "Thermic Effect" of food. In other words, to process calories, the body must use calories to do it. However the calories needed for digestion DOES NOT out-number the calories in the actual food being digested. This goes for energy drinks too. Therefore, whenever you hear an "expert" say; "Eating protein will jump-start your metabolism and cause your body to burn more calories", it is a misleading statement because although this statement is technically true - the "implied" message of burning calories above and beyond those in the food itself - is pure nonsense. Think of your Metabolism like the engine in your car. Your muscle, since they use the largest portion of your consumed daily calories, is like your body's ENGINE.

Your (Metabolism) ENGINE Works Like This:
0-5 mph: Idling at a Red-light but still burning calories.
(Just-like resting, sleeping, etc.)
5-15 mph: You're pulling out of the driveway onto the street.
(Just-like moving from room to room in your home, watering plants)
20-35 mph: You're cruising along on a residential road.
(Just-like housework, gardening, busy-body activities, office-work)
40-55 mph: You're cruising along on a flat open-road.
(Just-like brisk walking or manual labor, like raking leaves)
60-80 mph: You're cruising along on the highway.
(Just-like running, vigorous exercise, or intense manual labor)

The Moral of the Story: If you want "your" engine to burn MORE calories - move more, or move faster! If you want a BETTER burning engine, ADD MORE MUSCLE to your body! This is the only thing you need to know about your metabolism, because it's the only thing that matters.

"If" STARVATION-MODE is True, Where Are ALL The FAT Anorexics?

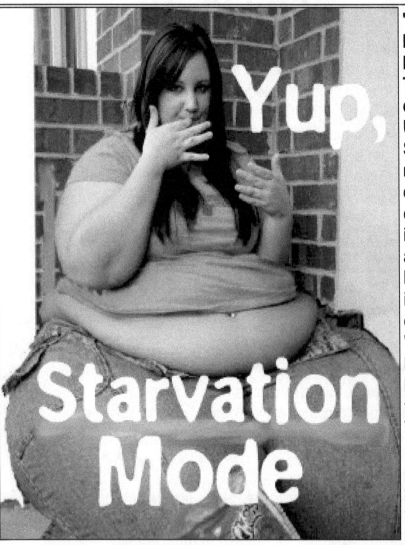

Yup, Starvation Mode

"If I Don't Eat Enough Food Each Day, Will My Body Go into STARVATION MODE, and Become Even FATTER?" Unfortunately, people STILL believe the common myth that the intake of "too few" calories will cause our bodies to go into "starvation mode", and therefore, since our body "thinks it's starving", it will then - as a means of survival - begin to "store instead of burn" body-fat. Eventually, you become another Starvation Mode victim; FATTER! Whenever I hear people say this, I always chuckle and ask, "If that's true, then where are ALL the FAT Anorexics?" Starvation mode is a myth that was popularized due to the Minnesota Starvation Experiment in which subjects were given 50% of their daily calorie intake for months. The result? Well, they lost weight until they had almost no weight left to lose and their bodies simply could not get the calories ANYWHERE. Concisely put: starvation mode happens when you are, quite literally, wasting away. Not when you have a simple caloric deficit. Your body will make up for it with fat stores. That's what they're for. Do not worry about Starvation Mode.

"If" STARVATION-MODE is True, Where Are ALL The FAT Anorexics?

Adding to that lunacy, you'll often hear people say, "The only way to get out of starvation mode, is to consume MORE calories to 'kick start" your now sluggish metabolism". Again, most people believe this, probably because they've have heard it so often, they guess it MUST be true. TRUTH: You cannot "eat more" calories to force your body to "lose weight". The laws of physics and thermodynamics will simply not allow it. Let's say a person claims to be eating only 1000 calories and not losing weight. A well-meaning friend then tells them that they are in starvation mode, and in order to lose weight they must eat more to "jump-start" their metabolism...okay...Then my question is, "What do you think would happen if instead a person just stopped eating altogether? Would they then go further into starvation mode and continue to stay at the same weight or maybe even "gain" weight?" Clearly, they would lose more weight if they stopped eating altogether. If Starvation Mode is true, shouldn't we be seeing anorexic people eventually become obese right before our eyes? Like many myths, this one is born out of semi-truths. There actually is a well-documented and true phenomenon known as the "Starvation-Response". However, it only happens in humans when they lose so much body fat that they fall below fat-levels essential for "survival". For men this would be below around 5%-fat and in women, just above that. This hardly applies to the average "Dieter" reading this post, or bodybuilders dieting for their next competition. My "Bodybuilding" friends usually like to jump in right here and say, "But, if we consume to-few calories we'll be burning muscle instead of fat, right?" Wrong again. This is another case of a slice of truth being blown-up into a major exaggeration. We always burn or lose some muscle (amino-acids) when we diet, no-matter how sensibly it's done. But, before it actually amounts to anything significant (or an amount that is noticeable in one's visual musculature), the body will first exhaust a LOT of its fat reserves. Bottom Line: If you are "over-fat" and NOT losing weight - regardless of your efforts to do so - the most important thing to do is re-evaluate your own "Energy-Equation". Yes, I mean "Calories-in vs. Calories-out". Outside of a special medical-condition, "weight-loss" will ALWAYS be the on-going balance of HOW MUCH YOU EAT vs. HOW MUCH YOU MOVE.

"Cellulite?" Is There Really A BEST Way To Get Rid of Dimpled FAT?

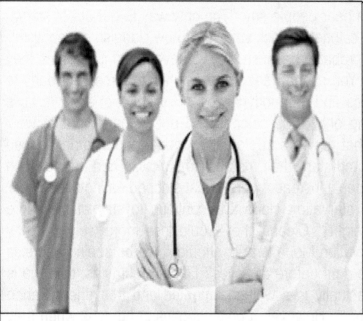

"Cellulite" A Women's Nightmare! What, if Anything, Can You Do about it?

Women dread the thought of looking down at their own legs, thighs, and butt, and seeing that damn DIMPLED and LUMPY formation of fat beneath their skin which resembles lumpy cottage cheese. Here's some facts you should know. **The Scam:** In 1973, a Diet-Book (What a surprise) by Nicole Ronsard, first coined the phrase "Cellulite". In a nutshell, Ronsard touted cellulite as a unique gel-like substance in the body. Supposedly, the only way to remove it was through various detox diets, massages, breathing techniques, blah- blah-blah. Nonsense of course! Well, the name stuck in the minds of women, and clever marketers have been cashing-in ever since. Americans spend millions each year on various magical creams, body scrubs, lofah pads, salon wraps, etc. The point? Stop wasting $$ on things that DON'T WORK! **The Truth:** Cellulite is no different than plain-ole body-fat. Most women experience this on their upper thighs and buttocks. The lumpy and dimpled appearance is caused by fibers of connective tissue in those areas which lose their elasticity with age. When body-fat pokes through this "grid-like" mesh of connective tissue, a WAFFLED and LUMPY appearance is the result. Sorry, the TRUTH is, there's not much you can do to stop it. Heredity can also be an influence. And NO, Cellulite does NOT contain toxins. **The Bottom-Line:** Losing excessive Cellulite is accomplished in the SAME way as losing ANY BODY-FAT, and that's by "Reducing Your Overall Calories, and Moving More". Yes, I'm talking about Diet and Exercise.

How Much WATER Do You REALLY Need?

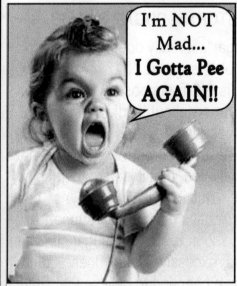

I'm NOT Mad... I Gotta Pee AGAIN!!

S--U--R--P--R--I--S--E!

The ole "Super-Hydration", and "Guzzle Tons of Water" folklore has made more than one expert shrug over the years. It's amazing how popular something with virtually no scientific validity continues be among close-minded fitness enthusiast. Proper hydration is important - nobody's denying that. However, seeing gym-rats carry around their bulky, plastic gallon-jugs of water is a little silly, and quite frankly, not supported by ANY unbiased scientific data. By the way, there is no such thing as "SUPER-HYDRATION." It's merely a popular bodybuilding fad. But hey, don't take my word for it. The best answer to how this myth started dates back nearly 70 years. The ole *"8-glasses-a-day"* mantra may have been the faulty interpretation of a 1945 Study. In 1945, the Food and Nutrition Board, now part of the National Academy of Sciences' Institute of Medicine, suggested that a person consume one milliliter of water (about one fifth of a teaspoon) for each calorie of food. The math is pretty simple: A daily diet of around 1,900 calories would dictate the consumption of 1,900 milliliters of water, an amount remarkably close to 64 ounces. Or, eight Oz. glasses - Mmm? At that time, many dieticians and other health practitioners failed to notice a critical piece of information from the research; namely, that much of the daily need for water could be met by the normal water content found in food. Dr. Heinz Valtin, a retired professor of physiology at Dartmouth Medical School, specializing in kidney research, and who spent 45 years studying the biological system that keeps the water in our bodies in balance, claims that the answer to the question, "Do we really need to drink water in excess of the normal amounts found in food, and dictated by our natural thirst?" - is a definitive "NO!" The good news is that there is little to no harm in drinking more water than is actually needed for good health. Toxic levels are extremely rare, even if you "tried" to drink too much. Excessive amounts of water will more than likely simply equate to extra trips to the bathroom. **It's interesting, the things people believe and the things that become popular in fitness and dieting pop-culture.**

The Little "White "Sugar Lie

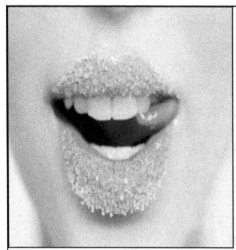

It is Time to STOP the SUGAR-SCARE!

Poor ole "Table Sugar"...it really does take an unfair pounding. Yes, I get it; sugar is NOT a "nutritious" food. However, it is NOT supposed to be...it's a freakin' sweetener for cryin' out loud! While I'm at it, you may as well digest another truth about sugar; it does NOT contribute to hyperactivity in kids. That myth is so widely believed, that it is hard to imagine that it's NOT true - But it isn't. There is not one shred of credible scientific evidence to support this too-common belief - look it up. Yes, sugar "is" for the most part, nothing more than empty calories. Yes, excessive sugar does contribute to tooth decay. I get it. The real point is that we have been led to believe that white sugar is "poison," and everything about it is evil. That of course, is nonsense. For all the "refined is bad" food-alarmist out there - get a grip. A teaspoon of sugar has only 16-calories, and compared to the alleged healthier-choices like raw sugar or honey, the truth is, they ALL end-up in the bloodstream, as glucose. Moreover, WHY do we care if it's sugar or high-fructose corn syrup in our soda pop? After all, we ARE talking about soda aren't we...not exactly a nutrition staple. Sometimes I think the "sugar scare" has MORE to do with marketing a more expensive product in its place (e.g., raw-sugar, artificial sweeteners, etc.) Sugar, like many other "bad foods," isn't actually "poison" at all. All things in moderation, right? By the way, sprinkle a little sugar on your bacon while it's frying in the skillet...it cuts down on shrinkage. By the way, giving up bacon would be a sin too...yummy! Eat what you want, and realize that it's the "rate of consumption" that gets you in trouble. In other words, a teaspoon of sugar here n' there = Good. 5-lb. bags of sugar per/day = Bad. A strip of bacon here n' there = Good. A pound of bacon per/day = Bad. I think you're getting the point. Bottom Line: We shouldn't be expecting table sugar to provide a great deal of nutritional benefit in the first place. **We should ALL be eating a cross-section of healthy foods to comprise our overall diet. Sugar is merely an accent-piece in the overall picture.**

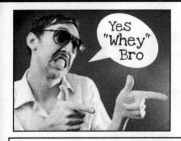

The Truth About "Protein Powder"

Question: "The Trainer at my gym says I should be drinking WHEY PROTEIN Shakes. Should I be?" **Short Answer:** Probably not. A well balanced diet with adequate amounts of lean meats or fish, low-fat dairy products, and/or various amounts of nuts, seeds, or legumes, will supply the body with all the protein it needs, and then some. **Longer Answer:** Should you use a Whey protein supplement? Maybe. Here's why: Mainly for convenience. Carbohydrates and fats make-up the majority of foods we eat; especially when we're grabbing something on-the-go. Protein on the other hand is a little less convenient to find in every-day foods without being laden with extra fat. Adding to the dilemma is the fact that it's just not practical to throw a steak, some eggs, or a piece of fish into a gym-bag or purse. Additionally, there are often refrigeration concerns - getting the picture? Whey protein-powder works in your body the same way a steak, eggs, peanut butter, cheese or dairy products do - but without the added fat-calories. Whey protein is low fat or fat-free, whereas a steak is not. Whey protein is a popular choice among protein supplements because of it being easily digested and assimilated by your body. Scientists call this "bio-availability." In addition, whey protein-powder mixes easily with most liquid without clumping. **Bodybuilders:** How much Protein should you be eating daily? The truth is, 35% - 45% of your overall daily calorie intake is plenty. Experts (the real ones) differ in their recommendation, yet most do agree on a number within this range. So don't micro-manage your exact %. Try to stay within this range - give or take - and you'll be okay. More Protein means Bigger Muscles, right? NO! This myth has been around since man first realized he "had" Muscles. Because the body uses dietary protein to make muscle, then more protein must mean more muscle, right? Wrong. More protein - beyond your needs - simply means more calories - period. Probably the BEST case you could make for taking a protein supplement is again, convenience. It's easy to whip-up a quick protein shake at home or carry one in your day-bag to consume during your workday. When it comes to understanding healthy eating and exercise, a small question often has a long answer. In an effort to keep this answer concise and to your point, I did not get into lactose tolerance concerns or the medical applications of whey protein or calculating protein intake, based on body weight. **Most people who INSIST that you should be drinking protein-shakes are usually SELLING them.**

10-Things I Should Never Have To Explain, Ever Again

1 - People Who Preform "Side-Bends" with a Dumbbell in Each Hand in an Effort to Trim Their Waistline, Are Dumbbells Themselves. (Simple Physics)

2 - For the Last Time...WOMEN Do NOT Get "BIG" From Lifting Weights. Women DO Get Big by Sitting Around Doing NOTHING too Often. It Amazes Me that this Weight Lifting Myth just Will NOT Die.

3 - CARBS Do NOT Make You FAT - Too Many CALORIES Does. It Doesn't Matter if it's Carbs, Protein, or Fat Itself, Eat Enough of ANY Type of Calories and You'll End Up Carrying it Around on Your Belly, Hips and Ass.

4 - "ABS EXERCISE" Do NOT Trim Your Waist. It's the BIGGEST LIE in Fitness. Yet, We ALL Start Doing More Crunches As Beach-Weather Nears.

5 - Protein Shakes DO NOT Cause Muscles to GROW Bigger, or Bigger Faster. Making a Muscle Work Harder than it is accustomed to, DOES.

6 - "Cleansing Drinks" and "Detox Diets" are For Suckers. Remember When "Experts" Told Us, We Each Had 5 LBS. of Undigested Red Meat in Our Intestines? The Joke was on us.

7 - FOOD Eaten Late at Night Does NOT Automatically Turn To FAT. Eating more calories than you burn DOES. No matter WHEN You Eat Them. Calories-In VS Calories-Out will ALWAYS be the Golden-Rule.

8 - ATTENTION MEN! Weight-Training Sessions lasting LONGER than 90-Minutes Are Probably NOT Intense Enough to be Most Effective. Train LESS, Train HARDER, and GROW Faster.

9 - FOOD Eaten Before Bedtime Does NOT Automatically Turn to FAT. You ARE Fat, Mostly Because You Eat Too MUCH, Too OFTEN.

10 - 2-Years From Now, CROSS-FIT, P90X, and "Functional Training Will ALL Be FADS Gone-Bub-Bye. They Will ALL Be Replaced By Some Other STUPID Thing the Clueless Will (once again) Fall For.

The MORE of These Statements You Disagree With...The LESS Informed You Are.

Chapter 5

FYI's, Q&A, N' Stuff

STOP Getting Advice From "They"

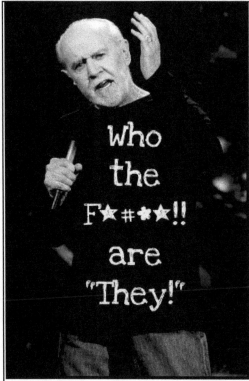

It seems like every time I hear somebody say something STUPID regarding Eating, Exercise, or Weight-loss, and then I ask, "Where did you hear that?"...
the answer I get most often is,
"That's what "THEY" say."

Famous comedian George Carlin once said, loudly:
*"They? Who the F**k Are "THEY!"...
And Why the F**k Do WE Believe Every F**king Thing "THEY" Say!...
WE Don't Even Know Who the F**k "THEY" ARE!!!!!!"*
As usual, just another one of George Carlin's brilliantly astute observations.

"They" are constantly advising us in our exercise and diet endeavors. Of course, "we" DO NOT speak directly to "They". "They" speak to us through others. There are hundreds of eating and exercise myths and misconceptions, constantly passed-on from one person to the next, and from one generation to another. Think about it, regarding eating and exercise, how many times in your own life have you heard someone say; "That's what "THEY" say". It usually sounds like this: "They" say you shouldn't eat late at night 'cause it turns to fat overnight." "They" discovered that green coffee can help burn body-fat." "They" say free-weights build bulky muscle and machines are for toning." "They" say you should exercise on an empty stomach because it causes you to burn more body-fat." "They" is often a euphemism for "A moron who really doesn't know what the hell he or she is talking about, yet they wanna sound really smart. Therefore, they just spew some "fact sounding" Bullsh*t your way and hope you're stupid enough to buy it, 'cause they don't have a clue. Always take what "They" say with a grain of salt. Better yet, just assume its BullSh*t, because it usually is.

My Personal Advice For Newly-Certified Personal Trainers

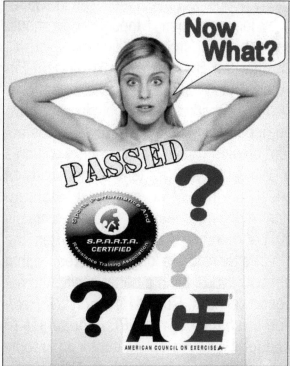

Congratulations, You've just earned your Personal Trainer's certification. Perhaps the most important thing for you to know at this point in your young career is the fact that you STILL know "NOTHING!" Ask any Real Estate Agent this question: *"After you received your Realtor's license, how much did you REALLY know about your trade?"* Answer: "NOTHING!" The same is true for any new and wet-behind-the-ears Personal Trainer. Moreover, "that's assuming" you became certified by an accredited and reputable organization. Lord knows there's an alphabet soup of organizations out there - both good and not so good. The responsibility is NOW on you to continue to be a sponge, soaking-up only factual or evidence-based training knowledge. Choose a mentor if you must. My opinion is that "High Intensity" Strength Training is the most evidence-based training protocol used by today's most informed Personal Trainers. That said, you should familiarize yourself with EVERYTHING out there. Part of your expertise is the ability to speak intelligently on any-and-all training modalities. Again, the educational process should NEVER ending Welcome to a fantastic industry and an exciting new trade. My hope is that as a NEW Personal Trainer, you will choose to be a part of what's RIGHT with this industry, instead of contributing to what is WRONG with it. A great start is to become familiar with the information on every page in this book.

FYI: Choosing The Right GYM to Join

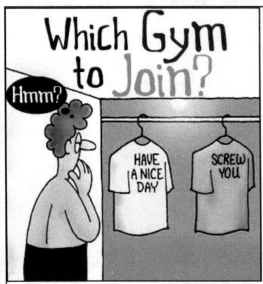

Since many people DO begin their "get in-shape" journey by joining a gym, I thought they should know a few things up-front. The first thing you will notice is that the Big Chain Gyms—Planet Fitness, Work-Out World, etc.—have taken-over most local gym markets - probably in your town too. The good news is that most mega-gyms actually "do" provide you with an incredibly valuable service. Which is, you get tens-of-thousands of square-feet of the latest and best exercise-equipment money can buy, all for approximately $10-$20 per-month - some even sweeten the deal with free tanning. As long as you realize that in most cases this is where the "cheap-goodies" end - you'll be in a better position to not be frustrated or waste money on other not-so-good services. **Rule #1** *You MUST Realize that Gyms are NOT in business to get you in-shape - Gyms ARE in business to SELL MEMBERSHIPS, Period!"* Take my word for it, offering ALL that they do for only 10-bucks makes "up-selling" other services and products a huge priority. You would have to be pretty naive to think that the weekly-meetings that take place in most clubs has anything with helping you become more-fit. Instead, it's an all-out blitz to train and motivate ALL staff to sell, sell, sell! Increasing-revenue is the ONLY meeting-agenda. To offset those low monthly fees the club is constantly brainstorming to create "additional revenue-streams." i.e. Personal Training, Supplements, Body-Composition Testing, Etc. Most of these services and products fall somewhere between "not-worth-the-money" and "a complete-rip-off". Are there exception? Yes. Personal Training can "sometimes" be a good value. However, when "unqualified" bobble-headed Barbie the Desk Clerk is taking-on clients for extra spending money, and the gym allows it, could there be a BIGGER rip-off! Read my "Personal Trainers" posts on my Facebook page before making any hiring decisions. I have always maintained that "good" Personal Trainers are usually under-paid and deserve MORE per-session than the current going rate. Moreover, the "Bad ones" give ALL Trainers a bad name. **Rule #2** *DO NOT EXPECT "5-STAR" SER-*

FYI: Choosing The Right GYM to Join

VICE AT MOST BIG CHAIN GYMS. Let's be fair and logical; You're paying $10-$20 per-month for a membership to a high-volume Mega-Gym Chain. It simply does not fit this particular business-model to offer enough floor-staff to cater to your every need (i.e. questions, advice, a "spot", etc.). Also, the Front-Desk Staff are - more than likely - under 20 years-old and often more concerned with texting, talking on the phone, goofing with other staff, or anything other-than a career as a Desk-Clerk Attendant. I guess you get-what-you-pay-for. **Rule #3** *Sometimes "free" really does mean free.* "Free" is usually a marketing-strategy used by clubs to get a figurative foot-in-the-door to SELL you something. The freebie that you really should consider is the "Free Introductory Session" with a Personal Trainer. Because the club or Trainer is hoping to turn the Introductory Session into a "sale" (i.e. Personal Training Sessions for a fee), you can usually count on the Trainer to be very attentive as they attempt to "sell themselves." Therefore, it is a great opportunity to pick-their-brain, ask them questions, get equipment demonstrations, etc. You really can turn this into a very informative session of great "tips" and exercise advice. After the introductory-session, the Personal Trainer will ask you to sign-up for paid-sessions. Unless you really think you need their services, politely decline the offer, thank them for their help, and say you are going to try it on your own. Do not feel guilty for "wasting their time". That is the cost of doing business. In fairness, "ethical" behavior goes both ways. If a club is a Personal Training ONLY facility, I believe it is in poor taste to waste their time hitting them up for a "free" session "if" you have absolutely NO intention of hiring their services. **Rules #4, #5, and #6** *(Things to consider other than price):* **LOCATION, LOCATION, LOCATION:** Is it a convenient distance from work or home? It's much more likely that you'll "skip-the-gym" if it's out-of-the-way to get to. Low membership-fees don't matter much, if you aren't likely to go regularly. **CLIENTELE TYPE?** It is generally more comfortable to be among group of people more "like ourselves" than not. Although it's easy to think it doesn't matter - it does. **NATIONAL CHAIN? or "HOMETOWN" GYM?** Although NOT always true, you can usually get a more "welcomed" experience from a smaller local-gym. The reason is that the manager is usually the "Owner". He or she may make customer service a higher priority than a lesser-vested revolving door Manager of a big-chain gym. Note: These statements are "generally" true. However, there are ALWAYS exceptions. Keep my guidelines in-mind, but use your OWN good judgment to make the best choice for "you".

"Functional Training" Really?

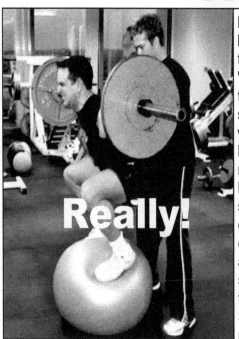

Really!

Remember SKETCHERS SHAPE-UP SHOES? No sooner had the science community exposed them as a foolish way to get in-shape, along comes another idiot fitness fad: "FUNCTIONAL TRAINING". Health clubs and gyms across the country are having a love affair this latest fitness nonsense. In a nutshell, Functional training is promoted as a way to strengthen your "Core" (another media-created buzzword), and improve your overall "balance", and, in-turn, making you stronger and better capable to perform "real-life" physical tasks, such as carrying groceries upstairs, stooping and bending while gardening, or plain ole house cleaning. The objective is to perform strength-training exercises in an "unstable" environment. So what! That stupid aforementioned SHAPE-UP SHOE actually worked on the same principle; it challenges your "balance" as you walk in them. Eventually, credible research exposed the Shape-Up Shoe as a marketing fraudulent product since it was determined that altering your natural walking mechanics was – for many reasons - unwise. Nonetheless, in gyms everywhere, we are now seeing Personal Trainers having people sit, stand, or lie on big inflatable exercise balls while performing resistance exercises. Again, the supposed value is that by creating an unstable environment in which the client must counteract, while simultaneously dealing with a particular resistance. Sounds good on paper, but the only thing it really does is prove that the Personal Trainer is a "dumbbell" themselves, and that the client is NOT using the best exercise protocol possible to accomplish what is probably their goal; to improve the way their body looks. Yes, you heard it here first: This form of training does not - to any great extent - cause improvement in overall physical fitness, muscular strength, muscular development, or body composition. Instead, it makes you look a bit silly in the gym, resembling a circus performer, instead of someone training in the safest and most efficient manner possible. ATTENTION ATHLETES! This faulty science is also behind much of the "Sports-Specific" Training that is being marketed not only to High School athletes, but athletes of ALL ages. Just know this fact: The best "functional" training for any sport, is the "sport" itself. We get better at throwing a football by throwing a football. Conversely, the only thing flipping tires makes us better at, is flipping tires. Make sense? By the way, I am NOT hating on functional training per se, I am against it being a mainstream first choice exercise application for your average person. These are the folks being ripped-off because it is NOT the best exercise protocol (not even close)... Nonetheless, it doesn't stop gyms from hyping it at the "next big thing!" Well, you heard it here first - it is not!

"CROSS-FIT"
Popular, But How Smart?

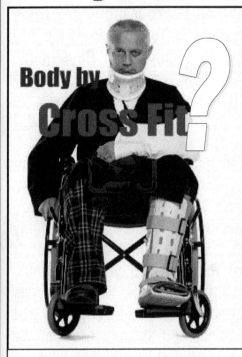

Body by Cross Fit

Is Beating the Crap Out of Your Joints REALLY Your Goal?" It may be time for "regular folks" to pump-the-brakes a bit before deciding on Cross Fit as their day-in and day-out workout of choice. Is Cross Fit a good thing? First, define "good thing"? My 1st thought: If you're engaging in Cross Fit to compete at it, or improve your specific ability to perform specific "Cross Fit" movements - Sure. In that case you'd be saying, "Cross Fit is MY "sport" of choice". However, if your real goal is to increase your strength or improve the way your body looks, you should NOT make it your "training-method" of choice. My 2nd thought: For those who regularly engage in Cross Fit - even if they're lovin' it, I wonder how their joints, ligaments, and muscles will feel, a few years from now. The bone-jarring, ballistic movements of Cross Fit are a lot like those in actual sports such as football and soccer. Ask Pro Athlete who has spent a good portion of their lives competing in such sports, how middle-age is treating them? Most can hardly walk normally, never-mind getting out of bed in the morning. In my own track n' field days, I lived on a steady diet of plyometrics, depth-jumping, and jump-squats. I shudder to think what my body would look like today if I continued to train this way to-date. My 3rd thought: I remember an old adage - "Do NOT Play Sports to Get in Shape - Get IN SHAPE to Play Sports." An effective strength-building workout should consist of slow controlled movements - NOT ballistic and joint-jarring routines. The goal of course is to better-prepare our body "for" the joint-jarring activities involved in sports. Bottom-line: Training is supposed to "strengthen" our body. Conversely, "Sports" beats the crap out of our body. That's NOT a bad or a good thing - for competitive athletes, it's simply the cost of doing business. I am NOT "hating" on Cross Fit. It what it is. In a new world of "EXTREME" everything. It appeals to a bad-ass, testosterone-driven, machismo that exists in many of us. Can you increase your fitness level doing it? Absolutely, but at what cost?

Don't Fall For
P90X®

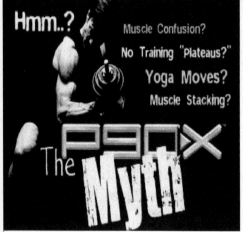

QUESTION: "My Husband Wants to Purchase the P90X Program Seen on TV. Your thoughts? Does it work? Do you agree with Tony Horton's Muscle Confusion Concept for Sculpting a Physique?" ANSWER: If you're really asking, "Will I have a sculpted body in 90 days?", My short answer is, probably NOT. As with most questions I'm asked, I usually end up circling-back to a few basic principles which explains "everything" to do with eating, losing weight, or becoming more fit. It's NOT that complicated. For starters, Abs exercises do NOT give you washboard abs. And, "Brazilian-Butt" moves do NOT re-shape your butt. There are many other posts on my Facebook page which illustrates this scientific fact. And please don't get me started on the dangers of the average-Joe doing P90X suggested "Plyometrics". P90X must provide a doozie of a "disclaimer" in their advertising to avoid "injury" lawsuits resulting from this joint-jarring exercise protocol. Furthermore, anyone who suggests that sedentary, overweight housewives would benefit from performing these-type of ballistic movements, is a moron! The proof that P90X-type Exercise and Weight-loss Infomercials are NOT telling the truth is ALWAYS found in the fine-print that accompanies such ads: **"These Results Are Not Typical", "Results Only Achieved When Combined With 8-12 Weeks of Reduced-Calorie Eating"** (Duh!). Often, the fine-print is the only thing in the entire ad, that's true! So, What about Tony Horton? He is the face of P90X. I am sure Tony Horton is a swell guy. However, his "real" genius is being an excellent "Marketer", NOT an Exercise Expert. For example, Horton's "Muscle-Confusion" and "Stacking Exercises" training principles are nothing more than "twists" on factual exercise science. "Muscle Confusion?" Sorry, muscles do NOT get "confused". Furthermore, what Tony Horton calls "Stacking", used to be called "super-sets", "giant-sets", descended-sets, drop-sets, etc. Marketers such as Tony Horton and ShawnT, simply keep inventing NEW words, or re-inventing old exercise terminology. Why? They have to, because if they didn't, there would be no "new" useless shit to sell you each year. Makes sense, right. My opinion is, Tony Horton probably knows the truth about his P90X, and the fact that the claims made in his P90X Infomercial are NOT reasonably accurate. Therefore,

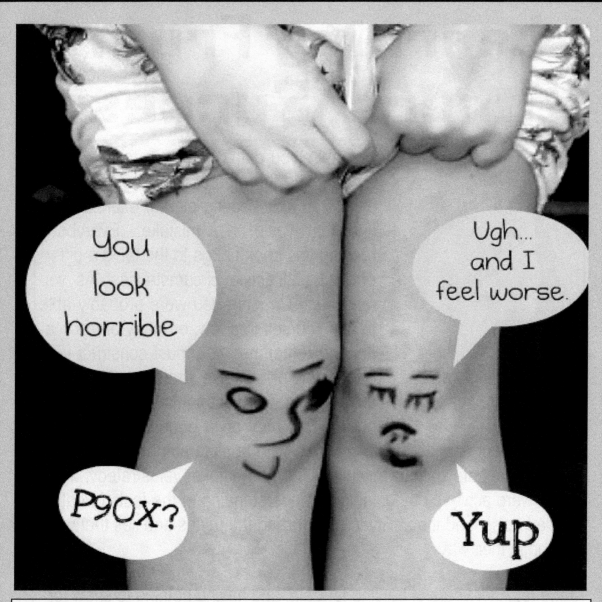

it's NOT a stretch to conclude that he is purposely misleading TV viewers. Hey, maybe any of us would in exchange for being rich for our efforts. Here's my bottom-line regarding P90X: Will it give you a good workout? Sure, if you perform the workouts regularly and religiously. By the same token, putting on a pair of grey sweatpants, an old beat up pair of sneakers, and then getting your ass moving, works too! P90X, in my opinion, is an injury waiting to happen; too many ballistic and joint-jarring movements for the average person - especially people who are "over-weight". I further believe that P90X has created MANY MORE disappointed consumers, than sculpted bodies. Take it for what it's worth. (P90X is a registered trademark)

Learning From Others' Success

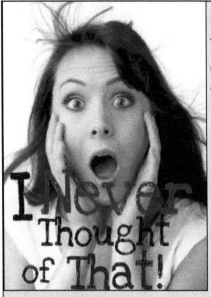

Hopefully you didn't just jump to this chapter, forgoing the others. This book does not dictate an exact eating-plan or exercise routine; that would be a mistake. Everybody reading this book brings to the table a different set of lifestyle circumstances. As you read each Chapter, you were probably able to find yourself in a few, or many of the scenarios. Remember, you must construct your own eating or exercise strategies by making the appropriate adjustments to your own lifestyle. This may be a good time for me to share a bit of experience from others who applied some of this book's advise to create their own successful body-makeover strategy. Their goals were achieved by gaining an understanding of the facts of eating and exercise, and the ability to recognizing the myths and lies that were getting in their way.

Janelle: After years of battling fat-gain, and having nothing to show for it except a kitchen cabinet loaded with half-full bottles of fat-burning pills and other weight-loss gimmicks, Janelle realized that product advertisements in soap-opera magazines were not the answer. Over the years, she purchased nearly every exercise gadget sold on late-night TV. These days, with a better understanding of what works and what doesn't, Janelle fast-walks for 30 minutes per day, and has given-up the stress-related bowls of ice cream that she sought comfort in.

Learning From Others' Success

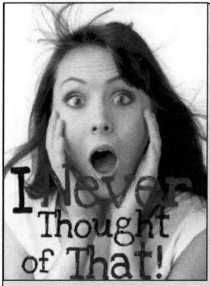

Ronda: After years of battling fat-gain, and having nothing to show for it except a kitchen cabinet loaded with half-full bottles of fat-burning pills and other weight-loss gimmicks, Ronda realized that product advertisements in soap-opera magazines were not the answer. Over the years, she purchased nearly every exercise gadget sold on late-night TV. These days, with a better understanding of what works, and what doesn't, Ronda fast-walks for 30 minutes per day, and has given-up the bowls of ice cream and other comfort-food snacks that accompanied her during the viewing of those late-night infomercials. She has lost 15 lbs. in six-weeks, and counting.

Amber: Amber is a former athlete who never paid much attention to calories. Also, because she always relied on a high activity-level and good genetics, her weight was never an issue. At 45 years old she wanted to take a closer look at her calorie-intake. After deciding on a "goal weight", and the calorie-intake to achieve her ideal weight, Amber used a 3-Day Food Diary to better understand how many calories she was consuming daily, and to get her on-track to eating the correct amount. After 3 days of tracking, Amber realized her average daily calorie intake was 3800. She made eating adjustments by cutting-down on the at work snacking, and using portion control in her daily meals.

Learning From Others' Success

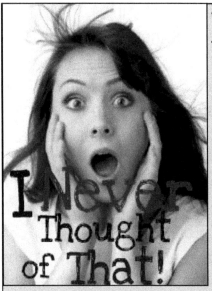

This allowed Amber to eat the same foods, yet cut her calorie intake to the 1600-or-so she needed to shed body-fat. She is currently at her goal-weight of 135 lbs.

Michelle: With good-health in-mind, Michelle switched from butter and margarine to healthier fats like olive oil. She then made a common mistake of thinking that because it's "good for you" fat, you can eat more of it. She soon learned, to her surprise, that ALL fat is the same calorie-wise. In other words, olive oil and bacon fat, although different "nutritionally", are equal in calories (9-calories per gram). She claims that this misconception alone was responsible for her recent weight-gain. She's back on-track, and is finding it easier to keep her weight in-check.

Megan: At 36 years old, she finally understood that taking an aerobics class 3 times per-week, wasn't enough to counter an overly sedentary lifestyle. At approximately 75 lbs. over-weight, Megan realized that by simply "moving" more, she was able to up her calorie expenditure over the course of days and weeks. Instead of camping on the sofa for most of her free time, she now engaged in more busy

Learning From Others' Success

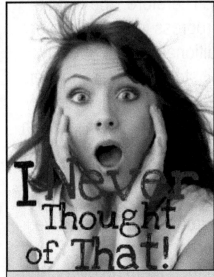

-body activities, like house-cleaning with her iPod playing her favorite 80's tunes. She parks her car in the furthest-away parking spot at malls and grocery stores. Megan finds way to add movement to her day. Without much change in her eating habits, she has lost 12 lbs. over the last few months. Not bad.

Wendy: (My personal favorite strategy) Deciding she needed to lose 20-30 lbs. Wendy remembered a magazine article I wrote regarding "Portion Control". It's one of the greatest weight control strategies around. She purchased an elegant set of dessert plates and tea cups. Without changing any of the foods she eats regularly, she served all her meals on these plates. Ice cream and creamy soups were only eaten out of a tea-cup. It made portion control a breeze. She still eats lasagna, pancakes, and all the foods she enjoys. The reduced portion sizes make cutting calories a breeze! Wendy went down 3 jeans sizes, in 3 months. Wow!

Linda: By adding intensity to her weight-training routine, Linda was able to add shapely new muscle to her legs and arms, all while cutting her actual time spent in the gym in half. She had been weight-training for years, yet never applied progressive resistance principles

Learning From Others' Success

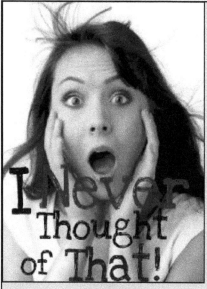

to her training. Therefore, she hadn't made much progress in her routine or body. The additional muscle not only looked great, it stoked her resting metabolic rate, resulting in overall fat-loss. She's now burning more calories, even while sleeping. Boy, the fat-loss value of weight-training...so under-rated!

Carrie: She purchased an expensive pair of designer-jeans, that were 2 sizes too small. She tried them on every Sunday morning. Motivated by the mere thought of having them fit comfortably, she committed herself to a new way of eating. Additionally, She begins each morning with a brisk walk-run through her neighborhood. Those "smaller" jeans can be a powerful motivator!

HERE'S MY ADVICE TO YOU: Re-evaluate your lifestyle. There is more than enough information throughout this book to dramatically jump-start almost anyone's your progress. Pick a strategy that will work for you. You know "you" better than anyone else, ever will.

My Favorite Questions & Answers

Over the years, I have answered many questions regarding Exercise, Fat-loss, Diets, Workouts, Supplements, Etc. Sometimes a particular question sticks in my mind and then finds its way into my blogs or one of my magazine articles. In this chapter I've selected a handful of my favorite questions. Many of them expose commonly believed myths and misconceptions. You may even recognize yourself in some of the scenarios. I hope you enjoy this "Questions & Answers" between me and a few friends I've met along the way...

Questions & Answers

QUESTION: "I want to know about "Creatine" for building muscle? Without a long complicated explanation that I wouldn't understand, can you just give me the bottom-line?" **ANSWER**: My short answer is that although studies have shown that Creatine does help to increase strength to some degree, it is STILL not a magic "muscle builder". People mistakenly believe that because some studies find it to be "somewhat" effective, they are ignoring that these same studies have called the benefits minimal at best. Building muscle is best achieved by following a high-intensity training protocol and hoping you have great genetics. Save your money for things that make more sense, like real food and entertainment.

QUESTION: "If you had to name the 3 biggest myths or misconceptions regarding weight-loss in 3 words or less. What would they be?" **ANSWER**: Ahhh, that's easy...
1 - Spot Reducing
2 - Abs Exercises
3 - Carbs Being Fattening

QUESTION: "I'm a Personal Trainer. Sometimes new clients will want to train in a certain way that I myself know is dumb. When they say, "it worked for my friend, why wouldn't it work for me?", I don't really know how to respond to that - are they right?" (I'm very frustrated - help!)
ANSWER: I am frustrated by this myself. Often people will attribute their weight-loss or exercise results to something "other than" what really caused it to actually happen. And of course it is hard to argue with *"hey, it worked for me!"* An example I always use is when people are hell-bent on doing set after set of sit-ups, crunches, and torso-twists to shape-up their mid-section. Of course, if they do see their waist shrinking in a few weeks, they never realize that it had nothing to do with all those needless Abs exercises. The other common example is when someone over-trains constantly, or always uses terrible form while performing weight training exercises, yet has an

Questions & Answers

impressive physique. Of course the reason is that it's "genetics" that has the biggest influence on how well, or not-so-well any person responds to exercise. In other words, a person who trains like an idiot, yet has favorable genetics, will ALWAYS get better results in the gym than a person who possesses poor genetic potential, yet trains perfectly. It's unfair, but true. The best we can hope to do as Personal Trainers is to educate our clients using sound exercise science and hope they're smart enough to "get it".

QUESTION: **"If you had to choose, would you pick low-carbs over high carbs as a diet strategy?"** **ANSWER:** I realize that "low-carb" dieting is very popular these days, but the truth is, a balanced diet that reduces overall calories is the smartest way to eat for otherwise healthy people. What good is low-carb eating if you are STILL eating more calories than you are burning. Extra calories make us fat - NOT the types of calories. It's incredible to me how many times over the years I have seen carbohydrates, protein, and fat, all take turns being the dietary "bad guy". If the weight-loss industry doesn't keep coming up with "new" ways of eating, they can't keep making billions, fooling us. It's that simple.

QUESTION: **"Has my metabolism really slowed down - and am I gonna get fat easier, now that I'm 40?"** **ANSWER:** Yes, and no. Your metabolism isn't really one tangible thing. It is actually the combination of every chemical-process taking place in our bodies. In regard to weight-loss, our metabolism doesn't really slow-down; we do. We tend to be less active as we settle into middle-age...that's the problem. But, what's really important to know is that after age 30-or-so, everybody begins to lose a small percentage of muscle-mass each year. This is normal and a natural part of our "aging-process." Muscle of course is very metabolically-active tissue, therefore, as we lose muscle, we will then get fatter on fewer calories than when we were younger. The good news is that we can offset much of this natural aging process with some form of weight-bearing or resistance-exercise. You can actually retain much of your muscle-mass and shapeliness as you age. The ole saying, "use it or lose it", really is true.

Questions & Answers

QUESTION: "**Which is more beneficial for fat-loss: building muscle or reducing calorie consumption?**" **ANSWER**: People have been told that building muscle helps burn more calories, and in fact, it does. However, between the two, "reducing calorie eating" far out-weighs any other factor in the weight-loss equation. This is why I hear people say, "I'm exercising religiously, but still not losing weight!" The reason is that they are not properly addressing their eating habits. Exercise can NEVER cancel out stuffing your face.

QUESTION: "**They say that cardio done first thing in the morning is good, as it targets only fat. Is this because the carbohydrate-reserves in the muscle are low-to-zero in the morning, therefore the cardio hits only the fat?**" **ANSWER**: No, No, and No. The body's fuel of choice is carbohydrates (converted to glucose and burned in the muscles). Fat is also burned in smaller amounts. We can not alter these percentages. As a matter-of-fact, in the absence of carbohydrates (glucose) our body converts amino-acids molecules into sugar-molecules. In other words, our lean muscle-tissue.

QUESTION: "**Why Do Bodybuilders "bulk-up" in the off-season?**" **ANSWER**: My Short answer is, because they're stupid! Although this myth of "off-season bulking-up" to add more muscle before you chisel it down via dieting has long died. Some knuckle-heads - mostly older guys - still believe it's the best way to get "huge". The truth is; off-season bulking-up should really be called off-season FATTENING-UP! After all, it would be a more accurate description. Much of this false notion has to do with the fact that as we get bigger (muscle and fat gain) we get stronger and feel "more" filled-out. Not to mention the thrill most muscle heads get out of seeing the scale jump up 30-50 pounds, and suddenly needing to buy an XXXL size shirt to fit over their now bulkier bodies. Therefore, I can understand how "bulking-up" seems logical to bodybuilders. But, it still makes no sense and has little to NO effect on the eventual amount of contest muscle you will have on-stage.

Questions & Answers

QUESTION: "I do a lot of crunches, cardio, and eat pretty-clean...why can't I get that last pound or two off my belly? It seems to be the hardest body-part to improve." **ANSWER**: Crunches will not burn fat off your abs, exclusively. The reason belly-fat (seems) like it is the hardest to lose is because it's often the body's biggest fat-depot. Therefore, as your fat-stores empty-out during fat-loss, the belly-area is often the last to be depleted, and experience razor-sharp leanness.

QUESTION: "You must see a lot of mistakes being made in the gym, I mean the way people lift weights. What are the most common reasons people are not getting good results?" **ANSWER**: Here's five simple things I have said over the years. I tell people to check themselves against all five, and if any apply to them - change!

1 - If it takes LESS than 20-seconds to perform a set of "any" exercise – the weight is TOO HEAVY.

2 - If you cannot control the speed of movement of a repetition to the extent that you could stop at any point if someone was to say, "STOP" – this means your "form" is not strict enough. SLOW IT DOWN.

3 - If you are spending MORE than 3 days per week in the gym, lifting weights – There is a better than good chance that you are OVER-TRAINING. Take MORE days off.

4 - If you perform more than 3-sets of ANY one exercise - then you have NO IDEA "what" intensity means. FIND OUT!

5 – Ask yourself, "Am I noticeably stronger than I was one year ago?" If "no", doesn't that give you at least some indication that something is WRONG with your exercise approach? FIX IT!

If you are GUILTY of ALL Five, it means you know next to NOTHING about "Weight-Training". However, now that you do know the truth, doing nothing to change would be just plain stupid.

Questions & Answers

QUESTION: "How many calories I should eat per day - all these sites and phone apps give me a different number?" **ANSWER**: The reason you get different #'s from different apps is because without doing complicated bio-testing, which is just a fancy way of saying your actual lean body mass, your total amount of adipose tissue (fat), your average daily calorie expenditure and a few other "lab" results, it is only possible to give parameters instead of exact calories needed. I like to say, "take your GOAL weight and then multiply that by 12". Again, just a ballpark, yet a good starting point. You can make adjustments as you go to account for variables and your own results.

QUESTION: "How many times/hours a week/day should I really be working out?" **ANSWER**: The short answer is "probably a LOT LESS than you think"...that's "if" you apply true exercise-science - most people don't. You don't specify if you are talking about weight training, Classes, or some other more aerobic-based activity such as walking. The more "intensity" used in your exercise sessions, the less frequently you perform them. For example: "Weight-training" should NOT be performed more than 3 times per week. Regarding cardio-type exercise, it can range from "the same as weight training", 3-times/per week, all the way up to 6-7 days per week being okay for very passive low-intensity walking sessions. Again, it's sort of a sliding scale when talking about "recovery time" needed to match the types of exercise sessions you engage in.

QUESTION: "I'm a professional musician and looking good/fit on stage is a definite plus. I do not, however, want to look like a muscle head. What's the best way to get nice and cut, without looking too bulky with muscle?" **ANSWER**: The truth-of-the-matter is; your genetics will largely determine your body's response to weight-training. I am usually asked this question the other-way-around, "How do I get bigger muscles?" To your question I would say, the answer is largely in

Questions & Answers

your eating-habits. "Leanness" is more a dietary-issue than an exercise-puzzle. Keep your daily-calorie-intake at approximately 12 x your goal-weight. For example: If your goal-weight is 175 lbs., your daily calorie-intake would be 175 x 12 – 2100 calories per-day. My 3-Day Food Diary is a great way to get an idea of your current calorie-intake-habits. Your exercise regimen could be cardio-based, however, I always recommend some-sort of full-body resistance-training. For you it could simply be a callisthenic-type-training – push-ups, pull-ups and such. This routine also works out well for traveling-musicians on the road.

QUESTION: "I'm a fairly active person; I either play disc golf, basketball, or go swimming just about every day. I no longer get winded or fatigued at the end of these activities anymore. Does this mean I'm no longer building cardiovascular strength? What should I do instead or as well?"
ANSWER: The reason you no-longer get winded or fatigued is that you have built-up a fitness-level that can easily handle your sports-activity. In-other-words, when summer began and you first started doing these activities, I'm sure you became easily winded. This is because it challenged your body's aerobic-capacity – another way of saying "out-of-shape". As you continued playing daily, you built-up your body's ability to handle – comfortably – these activities. To the last part of your question "I'm no-longer building cardiovascular-strength?" Actually, you're "maintaining" your new fitness-level. To build your fitness-level to an even-higher level you would have to increase the demands made on it. I'd say your fitness-level is already high. Relax – keep doing what you're doing – and enjoy the fact that you are now "fit!"

Questions & Answers

QUESTION: "I understand one set per exercise thing...but, should I also limit my-self to one exercise per muscle?" **ANSWER:** One properly executed weight-training set will stimulate the appropriate "adaptive response"
within a muscle. As you perform additional (same muscle) exercises, you get – at best – diminishing returns for your efforts. You also can make unwanted inroads to your recovery-ability (i.e. Over-training). As to the argument for working a muscle at "all angles," again, where do you draw the line? 1, 2, or 3, more sets? Even if there was a potential benefit, it would be incremental compared to the benefit of the initial set. Why spend hours in the gym if you don't have to?

QUESTION "Should I eat something small before I workout in the am? I feel like I lose weight better when I workout on an empty stomach but I'm starving in the am". **ANSWER:** The truth is, exercising on an empty stomach does not cause you to "Lose weight better" in of itself. That said, some people prefer to exercise on an empty stomach, and some prefer a small amount of food - preferably carb-type - in their system before a workout. It really becomes a matter of personal preference. Be careful; for some, the "no food" strategy can lead to an undesirable low-blood-sugar issue.

QUESTION: "I'm looking for a little advice on nursing and losing weight. This is something I never see anything written about. I'm assuming because of the need for extra calories?" **ANSWER:** In my opinion, weight-loss during a nursing-period-of-time IS possible. The important thing would be to reduce calories slowly and steadily - nothing too dramatic - and to keep nutritional density of the food you're eating, high. Presto!!! If a meal-in-a-can or a nutritionally-balanced food bar is quite desirable. These are a much healthier choice than the alternative, which is often grabbing a candy bar, a bag of chips, and a bottle of soda. A good protein-shake in a can will have 20+ grams of protein, 30+ grams of carbohydrates, and 1-4 grams of (good) fat. The food-bar should have approximately same ratio as the drink.

Questions & Answers

QUESTION: "I know that you say that 20-30 minutes of cardio is all you need in a workout. But, I simply love ZUMBA, and those workouts last roughly 45 minutes. Is working out longer than you recommend bad? I realize it may be "unnecessary" but don't care cause I just like it." **ANSWER:** My comments on cardio are with "efficiency" and "results" in mind. Can you perform "more," and get results? Sure! Say, for example, you do one hour of cardio each day, and get results from it. Assuming you have no recovery issues training like this...HAVE AT IT!

QUESTION: "Off the top-of-your-head, what are the two worse fat-loss products of all-time?" **ANSWER:** For Exercise equipment, I would say the "Thigh Master" promoted by Suzanne Somers. For Food Supplements, I'd say, "SENSA". You sprinkle it on food...and magically lose weight. Yeah right!

QUESTION: "Is there scientific basis to eating 5 meals a day 3 hours apart? Or does it matter as long as I get all those calories in somehow? I prefer eating every couple of hours to keep away the hunger pains, but other than that, does it matter?" **ANSWER:** The short answer is this; your weight-gain or weight-loss is a result of your calorie-in/calorie-out balance, over days, weeks, and months. It does not matter "when" a calorie is consumed. That said, even though the "math' would support it...it would be foolish to eat 2000 calories a day, in one sitting. The "3 meals", "five meals," when to eat, and how often, issue is a matter of individual preference. Unless there are specific "blood sugar" or "hypo-glycemic" issues in-play...Eat, drink, and be merry, whenever it suits you.

QUESTION: "If I Do My Cardio Too "Intensely", Won't I Be Out of My Fat-Burning Zone, and Just Be Burning (Only) Sugar?" **ANSWER:** This myth started in the 80's when we were told NOT to do our cardio or aerobics to strenuously because we would

Questions & Answers

NOT be in our "fat-burning-zone"...nonsense! Having a better understanding of aerobic and anaerobic energy metabolism would bear this out.

QUESTION: "Is Lifting weights is going to make me huge like a bodybuilder?"
ANSWER: Putting on muscle is not easy. It takes years of dedicated work. It is insulting to the people who do this on purpose to think you could get to the same level accidentally. Unless you're specifically training to "be huge" you're not going to accidentally get huge. And even if you find yourself getting bigger than you'd like, you can always stop working out to reverse these effects.

QUESTION: "In the gym I often hear much of the same advice over and over again. Do you have perhaps 3 or 4 TIPS that are either different or not so common?" ANSWER: Sure. Try these:
1 - When performing a set of any weight-training exercise, instead of "counting the reps", keep track of the time it takes to complete one entire set. Generally, if the time it takes to complete a "set" of any weight-training exercise is LESS than 30-seconds, you're probably a man - the weight is too heavy. On the other hand, if the time it takes is MORE than 90-seconds, you're probably a female - the weight is too light. 40-70 seconds is generally considered optimum for either sex - make the adjustment.
2 - The BEST way to develop "Six-Pack" Abs Doesn't involve "Picking Up" Weights or Dumbbells...It involves "Putting Down" Your Spoons and Forks. Make sense?
3 - Ladies, if your goal is a "better-looking body", know that the combination of weight training & portion-controlled-eating beats long sessions on the treadmill or group exercise classes - EVERY TIME! Nobody has EVER dramatically changed the way their body looks by jumping around in ZUMBA Classes 3 times a week. No really!
4 - We used to be told "exhale on exertion", and then "inhale while lowering the weight to the starting position". Although generally true, it may be time to slightly re-think that rule. Why? Today's smarter, more productive weight-training involves slower and longer repetitions; therefore, it becomes illogical to then assume that individual breaths

Questions & Answers

should now last up to 10 full seconds to coincide exactly with the repetition. It is now appropriate to also sneak short choppy-breaths during the movement to satisfy oxygen needs. You'll tend to do this naturally anyway, so just let your body breathe naturally, and stop over-thinking the ole breathing rule.

QUESTION: "Many times per year I find myself stuck in a hotel room with no workout facility available. I don't want to miss my usual "high intensity" workout. Is there anything I can do right in my hotel room that doesn't involve exercise equipment?" ANSWER: Yes, "Isometric" exercise. I'm talking about muscles working against an immovable force or opposing muscles. Most people do not realize that "full-range of motion movement", although favorable, is NOT a prerequisite for strength development. The "intensity of the contraction", and the "duration of the contraction" is the key. So yes, sitting and flexing your muscles can be productive work. In-other-words, strength and development can occur. For example: If you put your palms together at mid-chest level, with your forearm on a horizontal plane, and your elbows pointing east and west, then push each arm against the other. This is an isometric "chest" exercise. I would perform it this way; the contraction should be for a full 60 seconds. While looking at a clock with a moving "second" hand, begin pushing at (what you perceive to be) 25% of your strength, hold that for 15 seconds. Continue push, but for the next 30 seconds, push at 50% of your strength (you will begin to feel fatigue in the muscle), now, continuing to push...push at 100% of your strength (as hard as you can) for the last 15 seconds (it's going to burn baby... that's good! Remember to breathe normally throughout the entire 60 seconds). The reason I encourage the 12-30-15 second protocol has to do with avoiding injury. I have actually used this exercise method in hotel rooms, while vacationing (When there was not a gym available).

Questions & Answers

pushing at (what you perceive to be) 25% of your strength, hold that for 15 seconds. Continue to push, but for the next 30 seconds, push at 50% of your strength (you will begin to feel fatigue in the muscle), now, continuing to push…push at 100% of your strength (as hard as you can) for the last 15 seconds (it's going to burn baby…that's good! Remember to breathe normally throughout the entire 60 seconds). The reason I encourage the 12-30-15 second protocol has to do with avoiding injury. I have actually used this exercise method in hotel rooms, while vacationing (When there was not a gym available).

QUESTION: "How the hell does one break through a "training plateau?" It's so frustrating to see my progress stall or even go backwards".
ANSWER: This is really simple. Training plateaus are more accurately defined as "results" plateaus. Even when you do everything right, they are still inevitable from time-to-time. That said, if you are really stalling in your progress, the reason is most likely to be "over-training". In other words, too much exercise and NOT enough rest. The other could be psychological staleness resulting most frequently from a need to change things up or add some variety to your training program. Try taking a week off (I know it's tough), or totally switch-up your exercise sessions to reignite your passion for training. While I am on the subject, as difficult as it is to get people motivated to begin exercising, it is equally frustrating to observe "Gym-Aholics" who will NOT listen to the BEST training tip they'll probably NEVER try, which is to take a full 10-Days Off from weight training. I know, I know, you're afraid to lose muscle in the process. My reply would be, "Look, you haven't GAINED ANY in the past year anyway, what's it going to hurt?" "REST" will always be the most "under-used" training aid.

Questions & Answers

QUESTION: "I try to eat ONLY when I am hungry, but sometimes whenI do eat, I eat way too much. How can I avoid this from happening?" **ANSWER**: Eating ONLY when you are hungry seems to make sense, but I think for many, this strategy is actually backwards. Here's why: Whenever we feel hungry, it's usually because our body needs fuel. More specifically, we are actually experiencing a drop in our blood-sugar level. If you ignore this natural-occurrence and try to "tough-it-out" by not eating, you are being set-up by your body to overeat. The reason is that as you continue to put-off eating a bit longer, your blood-sugar continues to drop, and then you WILL over-eat! It's a natural survival mechanism. You suddenly become irritable, and eventually you'll let NOTHING come between you and food. Sound familiar? Your body over-reacts to hunger by gorging itself. Blame the cavemen for that. I'm not a big advocate of saying how many meals, and how often you should eat. I've known people who eat 5 - 6 small meals per day, and I know people who eat once a day, and it works for them - whatever. You know your body better than anyone. The folks that eat only one big meal per day are able to do this because they - for some reason - don't have a highly- sensitive blood-sugar chemistry (I'll spare you the complicated science jargon). Remember this: If you can get some food in your stomach before you get hungry, your body will be satisfied with a smaller meal. By getting in the habit of eating this way - therefore staying "ahead" of hunger-signals - you will probably have an overall lower daily-calorie intake because you'll avoid gorging. This may mean less fat on your belly, hips, and thighs.

QUESTION: "There are so many diets to choose from. Could you please tell me which diet you think is the best?" **ANSWER**: By now, most smart people understand that weight-loss really is a calories-in vs. calories-out energy equation - it's the Golden Rule of Weight-loss. Therefore, the secret to seeing your body-fat melt away is to simply tip the energy-equation scale in your favor by con-

Questions & Answers

suming fewer-calories. So, what's the easiest diet for most people to master? "PORTION CONTROL". And don't be fooled by its simplicity. It's a powerful and effective strategy, when done correctly. Portion Control is best, simple because it's the least restrictive form of eating. It's hard to stick to any diet that says you can only eat from a small group of food selections, or that "fat" or "carbs" are a no-no. When your family eats lasagna - you can eat lasagna too. Portion control and a little common sense will allow you to eat ANYTHING you want. You get to eat MOST of the foods you eat regularly by simply cutting the portion by 50%. Presto! Instant calorie reduction. Instant fat-loss. TIP: Never fill a large dinner-plate and then say, "I'll just eat half". It NEVER works. TIP: When dining in restaurants, ask for a "to-go" container at the same time you order your meal. When served, immediately put half of the meal into the container. It will be another meal, at another time. The BEST TIP: Purchase a few really fancy dessert plates. They're about 5-6 inches in diameter. Each time you eat a meal, serve it to yourself on these plates. It will naturally keep the portion-size down, yet have the appearance of a "full-plate." Breakfast cereals can be eaten out of smaller bowls or coffee-mugs, and foods like creamy soups and ice cream are eaten out of tea-cups. Get the picture?

QUESTION: "Will Losing weight improve sex life? What about penis size?"
ANSWER: Say What! Actually, I'm glad somebody asked it, and I'll give you the evidence based answer. YES! For overweight men with erectile dysfunction, small losses in overall weight (5 percent to 10 percent of total body weight in morbidly obese patients) DID improve erectile dysfunction and revived the ability to have intercourse. In addition, although the penis does not actually get larger (And don't fall for all those "BS" supplements and gimmicks regarding THAT whole issue...) the effective length will seem longer due to reductions in the perineal fat pad (the pad of fat just above the base of the penis.) When that pool of fat gets smaller, the "effective" penile length gets longer. However most studies show that effective intercourse has more to do with the mind than the size of the penis, since a large percentage of female orgasm is mental rather than physical. But that is a subject for an entirely different book.

Questions & Answers

QUESTION: "My Doctor sent me to rehab to strengthen my shoulder and arm after having a cast on for nearly 6-months. The "Exercise Specialist" I was assigned to must have been 20-30lbs over-weight... I was shocked! How on earth can they know ANYTHING about exercise if they are not in-shape themselves! Should I ask to be assigned to another Personal Trainer? **ANSWER**: This question makes me think of people in the gym who over-train constantly or who always use terrible form while performing weight training exercises, yet have an awesome physique. Of course the reason is that it's a persons' "genetics" that has the biggest influence on how well - or not-so-well - they (or anybody else) responds to exercise. A person who trains like an idiot, yet has favorable genetics, will ALWAYS get better results in the gym than a person who possesses poor genetic potential, yet trains perfectly. It's unfair, but true. If people are only willing to workout with Personal Trainers who possess the BEST physiques, then shouldn't we only go to dermatologists who possess perfect skin, dentist who possess the straightest and whitest teeth. And, in sports, if teams ONLY hired formerly great athletes as head coaches, then Vince Lombardi, Don Shula, Bill Belichick, Phil Jackson, and Red Auerbach would have NEVER been hired. If memory serves me correctly, didn't Magic Johnson fail miserably as a Head Coach, and Michael Jorden suck as an Owner/GM? ALWAYS choose your Personal Trainer based on the factual and evidence-based knowledge they possess; period!

QUESTION: "What do you recommend for an exercise routine? I currently go to the gym 3-4 days a week splitting my days into chest/shoulders, back/traps, and legs. I get what you said about reaching the adaptive response with strict form in sets lasting 40+ seconds, but I was unsure what a typical routine would look like? Also, would you advocate any cardio mixed in?" **ANSWER**: My answer to your question(s) would be this: Don't over-think any exercise or eating plan. Use the evidence-based eating and exercise principles only as the framework of the "plan" you construct for yourself. In other words, I myself like doing a modified push/pull routine: Day 1 - Chest, shoulders, triceps, quads and calves.

Questions & Answers

Day 2 - Back, traps, biceps and hamstrings. I choose - say - 2 exercises per body-part and perform only one set to failure. Pretty simple. I have also at times switched over to a full-body workout with 2 days off in between workouts. I adjust my workout routines to suit either my work-schedule or my current enthusiasm for training itself - which can ebb and flow throughout the year. Again DON'T OVER-THINK IT. Another important thing to remember is that there is NOT a "magical" rep-scheme or workout frequency that is going to make awesome results suddenly happen - when they have not previously occurred. In other words, we are ALL slaves to our own genetic potential. Most of us realize this potential - or close to it - after a couple years of engaging in even stupid workout routines. Supplement Ads suck people into buying useless products by claiming that this simple fact, isn't true. Sadly, it is. Regarding cardio? Let your own ability to recover be your guide. If you enjoy an occasional cardio-session; HAVE AT IT! Trust me, your body will let you know when you are over-training (if at all). Damon, I hope this helps. I'm sorry if I couldn't provide any brilliant "new" training secrets. There simply aren't any magic formulas to fast muscles or instant weight-loss. Keep up your great work!

QUESTION: "Would you choose good ole fashioned water, Gatorade or some other sports drink as your ultimate workout beverages?" ANSWER: This is going to surprise you, but according to nearly ALL the qualified health experts, the best thing to drink when your body is losing water is WATER. Sports drinks are packed with calories and sugar, which can be beneficial after an **extremely strenuous** workout sessions lasting an hour or more, during which the body loses lots of electrolytes. (which is just a fancy word for sodium and potassium) Most casual workout warriors are not taking part in that type of exercise, though, which is why the best thing to drink during a workout is water, and the best thing to consume after a workout probably is fruit or some other simple sugar - when the body is most receptive to replenishing lost glycogen (another fancy word for carbohydrates). I'll save you the long boring scientific explanation.

Questions & Answers

QUESTION: "Steve, I follow your blogs, and, I have heard you speak at workshops. You talk a lot about "weight-loss, diets and exercise". How did you figure this all out, and what are your sources for trustworthy and accurate information?"

ANSWER: I get asked that a lot. When people inquire about "my" expertise they are usually expecting to hear me talk about how I discovered a revolutionary new type of science, or invented a new "diet" or "training strategy", which I now claim would facilitate either faster weight-loss or bigger muscles. Nothing could be further from the truth. I am NOT smart enough to re-invent science. I have spent years studying mainstream peer reviewed science - as it applies to exercise and eating. I guess you could say I am merely a "Reporter" of sorts. I report on the accurate science of biological chemistry and physiology. It's the same information being taught in accredited colleges and universities. Too many people get their own eating and exercise knowledge from glossy magazines, "TV Personal Trainers" in infomercials, and popular gym folklore. All of which are NOT delivering on their promises to make weight-loss or ripped-muscles "fast, "easy" and "effortless". When people ask about my "sources" of information, I usually name the American Dietetic Association, the American Council on Science and Health, the American Journal of Clinical Nutrition, New England Journal of Medicine, American Journal of Sports Medicine, American Council on Exercise (ACE), the Harvard School of Public Health Information (A great Website), and the Mayo Clinic Public Information Website - another great user-friendly web-site. You don't have to know all the answers - just where to find them.

I HOPE YOU HAVE ENJOYED READING MY BOOK...
THAT'S IT!

References: My Proof & Evidence

Any book claiming to be factual or evidence-based should include credible sources of information for the claims being made. Here are the materials I used for the information and advice contained in this book.

"Cha De Bugre: Uses, Side Effects, Interactions and Warnings - WebMD." WebMD. WebMD, n.d. Web. 04 Dec. 2013.

Cloud, John. "Why Exercise Won't Make You Thin." Time Magazine 9 Aug. 2009: n. pag. Web. 18 Dec. 2013. <http://content.time.com/time/magazine/article/0,9171,1914974,00.html>.

Coffey, VG, B. Jemiolo, J. Edge, AP Garnham, SW Trappe, and JA Hawley. "Effect of Consecutive Repeated Sprint and Resistance Exercise Bouts on Acute Adaptive Responses in Human Skeletal Muscle." Am J Physiol Regul Integr Comp Physiol. 297.5 (2009): 1441-451. Web.

Coffey, VG. "Effect of High-frequency Resistance Exrcise on Adaptive Responses in Skeletal Muscle." Med Sci Sports Exerc. 39.12 (2007): 2135-144. Web.

"Correa v. Sensa Products, LLC Www.weightlosssettlement.com." Correa v. Sensa Products, LLC. GCG, 2013. Web. 18 Dec. 2013. <http://www.weightlosssettlement.com/>.

Dawson, Gloria. "Beer Domesticated Man." Nautilus. Nautilus. 19 Dec 2013. Web. 20 Dec 2013.

Feature, Elizabeth LeeWebMD. "Energy Shots Review: Do They Work? Are They Safe?" WebMD. WebMD, 28 Aug. 2009. Web. 04 Dec. 2013.

Fortman, Stephen P., Brittany U. Burda, Caitlyn A. Senger, Jennifer S. Lin, and Evelyn P. Whitlock. "Vitamin and Mineral Supplements in the Primary Prevention of Cardiovascular Disease and Cancer: An Updated Systematic Evidence Review for the U.S. Preventive Services Task Force." Ann Intern Med 159.12 (2013): 824-34. Print.

Fisher J, Smith D. Attempting to better define 'intensity' for muscular performance: is it all a wasted effort? Eur J Appl Physiol 2012;112:4183–5.

Philbin, John (2004). High-Intensity Training: more strength and power in less time. Human Kinet-

References: My Proof & Evidence

ics. ISBN 978-0-7360-4820-0.

"FTC Mails Refund Checks to Consumers Who Bought Skechers' Shape-Ups and Other "Toning" Shoes: Company Paid $40 Million for Refunds to Settle FTC Charges of Deceptive Advertising." FTC Mails Refund Checks to Consumers Who Bought Skechers' Shape-Ups and Other "Toning" Shoes. Federal Trade Commision, 11 July 2013. Web. 04 Dec. 2013.

Glenn, JM, I. Cook, R. DiBrezzo, M. Gray, and JL Vincenzo. "Comparison of the Shake Weight ® Modality Exercises When Compared to Traditional Dumbells." J Sports Sci Med 11.4 (2012): 703-08. Print.

Goodman, Brenda. "Experts: Don't Waste Your Money on Multivitamins – WebMD." WebMD. WebMD, 16 Dec. 2013. Web. 18 Dec. 2013.

Guallar, Eliseo, Saverio Stranges, Cynthia Mulrow, Lawrence J. Appel, and Edgar L. Miller, III. "Enough Is Enough: Stop Wasting Money on Vitamin and Mineral Supplements." Ann Intern Med 159.12 (2013): 850-51. Web.

Hall, Harriett, MD. "Defending Isagenix: A Case Study in Flawed Thinking « Science-Based Medicine." Defending Isagenix: A Case Study in Flawed Thinking « Science-Based Medicine. N.p., 22 June 2010. Web. 04 Dec. 2013.

Hall, Harriett, MD. "Isagenix Study Is Not Convincing « Science-Based Medicine." Isagenix Study Is Not Convincing « Science-Based Medicine. Science-Based Medicine, 11 Dec. 2012. Web. 04 Dec. 2013.

Hammer, Sebastiaan. Radiological Society of North America (RSNA) 97th Scientific Assembly and Annual Meeting; Abstract #SSE04-06. Presented November 28, 2011. SSE04-06. N.p.: n.p., n.d. Print.

Kroeger, Cynthia M., Monica C. Klempel, Surabi Bhutani, John F. Trepanowski, Christine C. Tangney, and Krista A. Varady. "Improvement in Coronary Heart Disease Risk Factors during an Intermittent Fasting/calorie Restriction Regimen: Relationship to Adipokine Modulations." Nutrition and Metabolism. Nutrition and Metabolism, 2012. Web. 4 Dec. 2013.
Nutrition & Metabolism 2012, 9:98

Fry AC. The role of resistance exercise intensity on muscle fibre adaptations. Sports Med 2004;34:663–79. Willardson JM, Burkett LN. The effect of different rest intervals between sets on vol-

References: My Proof & Evidence

ume components and strength gains. J Strength Cond Res 2008;22:146–52.

Lamas, Gervasio A., Robin Boineau, Christine Goertz, Daniel Mark, Yves Rosenberg, Mario Styliano, Theodore Rozema, Richard Nahim, Lauren Lindblad, Eldrin Lewis, Jeanne Drisco, and Kerry Lee. "Oral High-Dose Multivitamins and Minerals After Myocardial Infarction: A Randomized Trial." Annals of Internal Medicine. N.p., 16 Dec. 2013. Web. 18 Dec. 2013. <http://annals.org/article.aspx?articleid=1789248>.

Lee, Elizabeth. "Energy Shots Review: Do They Work? Are They Safe?" WebMD. WebMD, 2013. Web. 18 Dec. 2013. <http://www.webmd.com/food-recipes/features/energy-shots-review>.
Leith, William. "Evolution Makes Us Fat." The Telegraph. Telegraph Media Group, 27 Sept. 2007.

 Web. 18 Dec. 2013. <http://www.telegraph.co.uk/culture/books/non_fictionreviews/3668156/Evolution-makes-us-fat.html>. Lewis, Alwin C. Why Weight Around?: Changing the Weight Loss Strategy. S.L.: S.N., 2007. Print

Hatfield, Frederick C. "Is High Intensity Training Best?". Dr. Weitz Chiropractic and Rehabilitation. Retrieved 2008-10-17.

Jump up ^ Carpinelli, Ralph N.; Otto, Robert M.; Winett, Richard; (June 2004). "A critical analysis of the ACSM position stand on resistance training: Insufficient evidence to support recommended training". Journal of Exercise Physiology online 7 (3). ISSN 1097-9751. Retrieved 2007-07-01.

McDonagh, M. JN, and C. TM Davies. "Adaptive Response of Mammalian Skeletal Muscle to Exercise with High Loads." European Journal of Applied Physiology and Occupational Physiology 52.2 (1984): 139-55. Print.

Miller, Anna. "Popular but Dangerous: 3 Vitamins That Can Hurt You." US News. U.S.News & World Report, 24 Feb. 2012. Web. 18 Dec. 2013. <http://health.usnews.com/health-news/diet-fitness/articles/2012/02/24/popular-but-dangerous-3-vitamins-that-can-hurt-you>.

Kirschbaum C, Pirke KM, Hellhammer D. The 'Trier Social Stress Test'—a tool for investigating psychobiological stress responses in a laboratory setting. Neuropsychobiology 1993;28:76–81.

 Kristensen J, Franklyn-Miller A. Resistance training in musculoskeletal rehabilitation: a systematic review. Br J Sports Med 2012;46:719–26.

References: My Proof & Evidence

Carpinelli R, Otto RM, Winett RA. A critical analysis of the ACSM position stand on resistance training: insufficient evidence to support recommended training protocols. J Exerc Physiol 2004;7:1–60.

Fisher J, Steele J, Bruce-Low S, et al. Evidence-based resistance training recommendations. Med Sport 2011;15:147–62.

Steele J, Fisher J, McGuff D, et al. Resistance training to momentary muscular failure improves cardiovascular fitness in humans: a review of acute physiologicalresponse and chronic physiological adaptations. J Exerc Physiol 2012;15:53–80.

Hoeger WWK, Hopkins DR, Barette SL, et al. Relationship between repetitions and selected percentages of one repetition maximum: a comparison between untrained and trained males and females. J Strength Cond Res 1990;4:46–54.

Shimano T, Kraemer WJ, Spiering SA, et al. Relationship between the number of repetitions and selected percentages of one repetition maximum in free weight exercises in trained and untrained men. J Strength Cond Res 2006;20:819–23.

Carpinelli R. The size principle and a critical analysis of the unsubstantiated heavier-is-better recommendation for resistance training. J Exerc Sci Fitness 2008;6:67–86.

Swart J, Lindsay TR, Lambert MI, et al. Perceptual cues in the regulation of exercise performance—physical sensations of exercise and awareness of effort interact as separate cues. Br J Sports Med 2012;46:42–8.

Helmhout PH, Harts CC, Staal JB, et al. Comparison of a high-intensity and a low-intensity strengthening training program as minimal intervention treatment in low back pain: a randomized trial. Eur Spine J 2004;13:537–47.

Harts CC, Helmhout PH, de Bie RA, et al. A high-intensity strengthening program is little better than a low-intensity program or a waiting listcontrol group for chronic low back pain: a randomised clinical trial. Aust J Physiother 2008;54:23–31. Steele

Goodman, Brenda. "Weight Loss Improves Erections in Obese Men With Diabetes." Medscape.com. Medscape, 10 Aug. 2011. Web. 19 Dec. 2013. <http://www.medscape.com/

References: My Proof & Evidence

viewarticle/747825>.

Izquierdo M, Ibanez J, Gonzalez-Badillo JJ, et al. Differential effects of strength training leading to failure versus not to failure on hormonal responses, strength, and muscle power gains. J Appl Physiol. 2006;100:1647–1656.

Kramer J, Stone M, O'Byrant H, et al. Effects of single vs multiple sets of weight training. Impact of volume, intensity and variation. J Strength Cond Res. 1997;11:143–147.

Hicks AL, Kent-Braun J, Ditor DS. Sex differences in human skeletal muscle fatigue. Exerc Sport Sci Rev. 2001;29:109–112.

National Strength and Conditioning Association. Essentials of Strength Training and Conditioning. Champaign, IL: Human Kinetics; 2000.

Fry AC. The role of resistance exercise intensity on muscle fibre adaptations. Sports Med. 2004;34:663–679.

Kraemer WJ, Ratamess NA. Fundamentals of resistance training: progression and exercise prescription. Med Sci Sports Exerc. 2004;36:674–688.

Linnamo V, Pakarinen A, Komi PV, Kraemer WJ, Hakkinen K. Acute hormonal responses to submaximal and maximal heavy resistance and explosive exercises in men and women. J Strength Cond Res. 2005;19:566–571.

Bishop PA, Jones E, Woods AK. Recovery from training: a brief review: brief review. J Strength Cond Res. 2008;22:1015–1024.

Salmon, S., and J. Henriksson. "The Adaptive Response of Skeletal Muscle to Increased Use." Muscle Nerve 4 (1981): 94-105. Print.

"Sensa Weight Loss Class Action Settlement." Sensa Weight Loss Class Action Settlement. N.p., 17 Sept. 2012. Web. 04 Dec. 2013.

"Sensa Weight Loss System - Official Site - Lose Weight with Sensa." Sensa Weight Loss System - Official Site - Lose Weight with Sensa. N.p., n.d. Web. 04 Dec. 2013.

References: My Proof & Evidence

Shaun T's Miracle 15-Minute Workout." The Dr. Oz Show. The Dr. Oz Show, 15 Feb. 2012. Web.

Siri-Tarino, P. W., Q. Sun, F. B. Hu, and R. M. Krauss. "Meta-analysis of Prospective Cohort Studies Evaluating the Association of Saturated Fat with Cardiovascular Disease." American Journal of Clinical Nutrition 91.3 (2010): 535-46. Print.

Stiles, Steve. "Bariatric Surgery in Type 2 Diabetes: Half in Complete or Partial Remission at 6 Years." Medscape.com. Medscape, 26 Apr. 2013. Web. 19 Dec. 2013. <http://www.medscape.com/viewarticle/803189>.

Stiles, Steve. "Low-Glycemic Diet Seen to Reverse Diastolic Dysfunction of Diabetes." Medscape.com. Medscape, 23 Apr. 2013. Web. 19 Dec. 2013. <http://www.medscape.com/viewarticle/802947>.

Zieman, E., T. Grzywacz, M. Luszczyk, R. Laskowski, RA Olek, and AL Gibson. "Aerobic and Anaerobic Changes with High-intensity Interval Training in Active College-aged Men." J Strength Cond Res. 25.4 (2011): 1104-112. Print.

Author Bio: Steve Gallagher

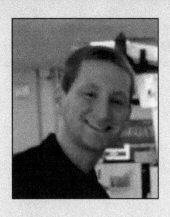

Steve Gallagher is an innovative and often controversial writer. Nonetheless, he offers no apology for ruffled feathers or raised eyebrows within the billion-dollar Fitness and Weight-loss Industry. Gallagher continues to be an aggressive advocate against frauds and scams propagated by - as he puts it - "an industry's shamelessly selling false hope to a mostly uninformed public." He studied Personal Training/Nutrition and is certified by the National Personal Training Institute, the premiere personal training school in the United States. Gallagher often credits an early-age fascination with working out for igniting his passion for uncovering the "real" science of nutrition, exercise, and athletic-performance improvement. In 2012 he formed the personal training/nutrition company, "Celebration Fitness," as he says, "there is a HUGE void in the industry. He continues to keep the public informed and protect everybody from myths, lies, and industry nonsense." In 2013, his first book titled, "Evidence Based Dieting, Exercise & Weight-Loss," became an instant internet hit. Steve Gallagher continues his efforts to improve the Personal Training industry by encouraging Trainers to make a commitment to their client's "Results" by implementing sound eating and exercise principles, instead of gimmicky exercise protocols and useless dietary supplements. Currently a Fitness Expert and writer, Steve Gallagher's latest project has him teamed-up with good friend, Franny Goodrich and Dr. Arthur Apolinario, MD. The three have collaborated on the 2014 book, "The Last Diet, Exercise, & Weight-loss Book You Will EVER Need to Read," as well as the development of educational workshops and personal trainer development. Steve Gallagher currently resides in Philadelphia, Pennsylvania. He can be contacted at Steve@celebrationfit.com

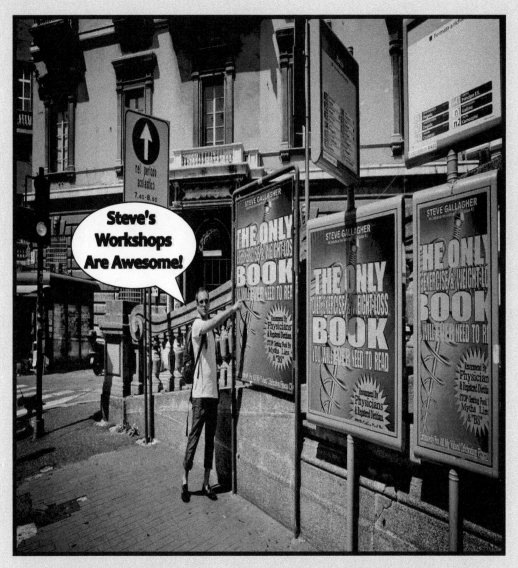

Printed in the USA
CPSIA information can be obtained
at www.ICGtesting.com
LVHW070537210124
769526LV00014B/1065